W9-CSZ-390

NATURAL HEALTH
AND BEAUTY

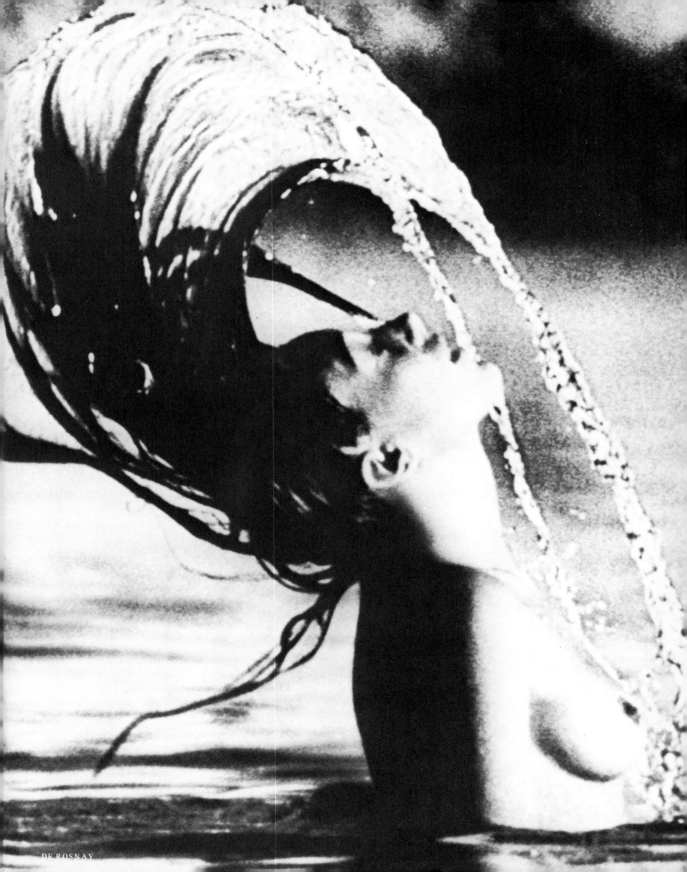

DE ROSNAY

BRONWEN MEREDITH

NATURAL HEALTH AND BEAUTY

Holt, Rinehart and Winston
New York

For Arabella

Copyright © 1979 by Bronwen Meredith.
Illustrations copyright © 1916 (renewed 1944), 1917 (renewed 1945), 1918 (renewed 1946), 1919 (renewed 1947), 1920 (renewed 1948), 1921 (renewed 1949), 1922 (renewed 1950), 1923 (renewed 1951), 1924 (renewed 1952), 1925 (renewed 1953), 1926 (renewed 1954), 1927 (renewed 1955), 1928 (renewed 1956), 1929 (renewed 1957), 1930 (renewed 1958), 1931 (renewed 1959), 1932 (renewed 1960), 1933 (renewed 1961), 1934 (renewed 1962), 1935 (renewed 1963), 1936 (renewed 1964), 1937 (renewed 1965), 1938 (renewed 1966), 1939 (renewed 1967), 1940 (renewed 1968), 1941 (renewed 1969), 1942 (renewed 1970), 1943 (renewed 1971), 1944 (renewed 1972), 1945 (renewed 1973), 1946 (renewed 1974), 1947 (renewed 1975), 1948 (renewed 1976), 1949 (renewed 1977), 1950 (renewed 1978), 1951 (renewed 1979), 1952 (renewed 1980), 1953 (renewed 1981), 1954, 1955, 1956, 1957, 1958, 1959, 1960, 1961, 1962, 1963, 1964, 1965, 1966, 1967, 1968, 1969, 1970, 1971, 1972, 1973, 1974, 1975, 1976, 1977, 1978, 1979 by The Condé Nast Publications Ltd.

All rights reserved, including the right to reproduce
this book or portions thereof in any form.

First published in the United States in 1981 by
Holt, Rinehart and Winston, 383 Madison Avenue, New York, New York 10017.
Originally published in Great Britain under the title
Vogue Natural Health and Beauty in 1979.
Library of Congress Cataloging in Publication Data
Meredith, Bronwen.
    Natural health and beauty.
British ed. published in 1977 under title: Vogue
body and beauty book.
    Includes index.
I. Beauty, Personal.   2. Women — Health and hygiene.
I. Title.
RA778.M487 1981   646.7′2′088042   80-26030
ISBN 0-03-057976-7

First American Edition

Designed by Paul Bowden
Drawings: Plants by George Suter; exercises by Rosalyn Toohig

Set in Monophoto Photina by Filmtype Services Limited, Scarborough, U.K.

Colour separations by Culvergraphics, Lane End, Buckinghamshire, U.K.

Printed in the United States of America
10 9 8 7 6 5 4 3 2 1

PART I HEALTH AND ENERGY

PART II POWER OF PLANTS

PART III BEAUTY PREPARATIONS

PART IV HEALTHY EATING

In writing this book I would like to express my appreciation to Alex Kroll, editor of Condé Nast Books who directed throughout and selected the illustrations, Barbara Tims of *Vogue*, Jacqueline Cattermole of Condé Nast Books, Eleo Gordon and Esther Sidwell of Allen Lane/Penguin Books, Judy Allen, who assisted in the cooking section, and Rhana Slett, who assisted me in everything.

FOREWORD

Good health and radiant looks depend on a multitude of factors including heredity, environment, your mental and spiritual attitude to life . . . but they also depend on one's awareness of natural resources and one's ability to make the best use of them. Healing power is present in all living things, and to realize this is to become conscious of an energy process that puts us in harmony with our environment. It is not so much going back to nature, but looking at it through enlightened eyes, for we judge its value against the claims of science. The idea of bringing the body to its optimum level of health the natural way is appealing and challenging. It is the ultimate of self-motivation. It is also logical, for if animals can control their metabolic conditions, why can't we. We have lost the instinct, the direct contact with nature; we have to be taught again. The natural approach to health and beauty is made on all levels: it is an adjustment in dieting and eating, a balance in structure, breathing and movement, a mental contact with the cosmic forces, a knowledge of the elements and plant life. This book provides a basis for the rediscovery of the naturally healthy body.

A word of precaution: self-diagnosis and self-healing are not advocated when an illness is obvious. If you are sick, see a licensed medical practitioner. No diet régime should commence without medical approval.

PART I HEALTH

ARTHUR ELGORT

AND ENERGY

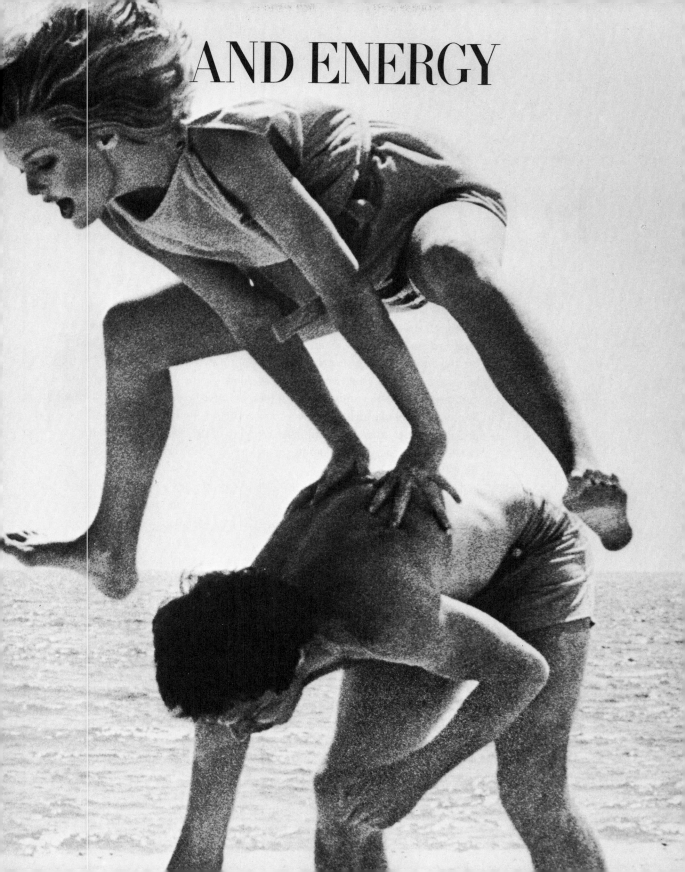

1

FOOD FACTS

Most of us are eating too much food and too much of the wrong food. Although the relationship between food and health is established, there is little agreement as to the extent of its influence. We have been brainwashed by the food industry and by the now outdated nutrition theory into believing that all that we need from food is the elements – protein, carbohydrates, fats, vitamins and minerals – regardless of their source. This limited concept of nutrition is based purely on the chemical analysis of food and does not take into account the interplay of these elements in natural foods, nor the complexities of interaction in the body, nor the possibility of nutrients yet undiscovered.

There is no substitute for natural fresh food. The body is not a machine that works no matter what type or quality of power you put into it; every body is unique in its nutritional requirements, which depend on biological, social and emotional forces.

Look at it this way: a great part of our diet is now convenience food – canned, frozen and instant concoctions that are easy to prepare. It is food that has been pulled apart and reassembled with synthetic elements. There are additives to give colour, taste, sparkle and smell, and preservatives to give the food a long shelf life. The final cost of a diet based on such foods will not be known for several generations, but the possible genetic dangers are already causing concern. A major problem is that many nutritionists have not caught up with the advances made in the understanding of cell and molecular biology, while the food industry is reluctant to accept that the fundamentals of mass commercial food production might be nutritionally and ecologically unsound. It justifies its position by saying that it would be impossible to produce the quantity and type of food demanded without the use of its processing technology or additives.

On a personal level, play safe and avoid processed foods as much as possible; work out a formula that meets the dual demands of healthy eating and of established eating habits. It is not at all easy to suddenly reform one's diet; to change to improve one's general health needs discipline.

We have almost got into the habit of living to eat rather than vice versa. Our lives are invariably organized around meal times and many social functions and celebrations are associated with eating.

A fault in nutrition can adversely affect the mind as well as the body, leading to lethargy, irritability and depression. By the same token, a faulty attitude towards nutrition can make you ignore wholesome food and neglect completely the basic requirements your body needs. The psychology of eating involves four principles.

Hunger: This is a prime urge that indicates eating is necessary. Few people in western societies know the feeling of real hunger pains. However, the more you eat the more the stomach expands and the more you need to eat. You experience pangs of hunger, but this does not mean the body is starving for food – simply that it is ready for more. Most people could easily live off stored fat and other matter for a few days or more – as during fasting – and the body would stop sending out automatic hunger signals to the brain, until such time as reserve supplies had been consumed.

Appetite: This is a tendency to eat that is present even if you are not really hungry. The brain centre which regulates this is called the appestat and some scientists believe that its abnormal functioning is responsible for over-eating and obesity. Appetite is stimulated by taste, smell, sight and touch of food. Colour is one of the most significant influences and we make conscious or subconscious decisions on what looks appetizing before we try it for flavour and texture. Red stimulates the appetite, orange is enticing, yellow has a favourable effect but only when bright or strong and earthy, not pale; clear rich greens represent freshness; browns are now associated with goodness, due to the influence of the health shops and their products. But take care; these are the very colours that are added to processed foods (even many brown breads are coloured to look more natural).

Habit: This is probably the strongest influence in the choice of food. We are inclined to continue eating more or less the same things for years, if not a lifetime. Habits invariably date back to childhood, when the eating plan of the family was adopted. The early association of ice-cream, cakes and creamy puddings as special treats is often firmly entrenched. Adopting new and healthy habits is difficult; let it be a challenging adventure.

Custom: We are not only creatures of habit but followers of custom. We are conditioned to eat the food of the society we live in; to differ from the crowd is often awkward for it can affect social activities, which revolve around eating. It is, however, not difficult to select wholesome food from the wide range of fresh produce available and cook and serve it according to the social convention. Nor is it difficult to pick out the healthy dishes from a restaurant menu.

In general, these principles have often been abused. The result is a society that is overweight and not nearly as healthy as it could be. This is primarily due to the over-emphasis on refined carbohydrates (sugars, flours, grains, cereals) in western diets. It is now believed that this is responsible for many body disorders, and that changes in eating habits over the last century have seriously upset the balance of the whole organism. For example, in 150 years the amount of sugar we consume per head has jumped eightfold from a reasonable fifteen pounds a year to 123 pounds.

The result of this indulgence in refined sugar and flour is not only overweight, but a whole range of other conditions; the relationship between the consumption of refined carbohydrates and the loss of teeth is obvious; diabetes is now being considered in this context, as the pancreas, which deals with sugar metabolism, suffers when it has to deal with excess carbohydrates of the sugary-starch kind; other consequences include unnatural loading of the colon, gall bladder and kidney troubles, coronary disease and stomach disorders. There is a significant increase in the occurrence of ulcers in the stomach and in the duodenum in people who eat processed food as compared with those who live on unrefined food.

A good diet not only maintains health, promotes growth and provides energy, it is also our chief natural protection against disease. Antibodies, for example, which are produced in our blood to protect us against bacterial and virus disease, require the availability of certain amino acids which come from the protein in our diet. We can subsist on bad food but resistance to disease is impaired and built-in therapeutic sources are depleted. It is the quality and compound composition of the essential nutrients that matter. Foods vary in what they provide, but if we select from the full range of natural foods, we can more than cover our requirements. (For details on the necessary nutrients, their source and value, see Food Values, page 225ff.)

There is a great deal of controversy regarding the difference and the usefulness of synthetic versus natural vitamins. Natural therapists usually claim that synthetic vitamins are ineffective and could be harmful;

orthodox doctors and nutritionists say that because synthetic vitamins have an identical molecular chemical structure, they are equally effective. Whom should we believe?

As a rule it is always better to trust nature. There is not enough evidence to support one claim rather than the other. It must be remembered, however, that our knowledge of vitamins is not complete and that in nature vitamins are never isolated, but emerge as vitamin complexes. When you balance natural foods you are getting all the vitamins that occur naturally; with synthetic substitution there is a chance that you may be missing out on a part that has not yet been discovered. Vitamins for preventive and maintenance purposes should be taken in foods and juices (see pages 17–19), or in complete supplements such as brewer's yeast, rose hips, kelp, herbs, nuts and vegetable oils. If isolated vitamins are necessary, it is wise to read the labels to find out which come from natural sources and which do not. There is no specific guide but, as a rule, if the label does not say that the vitamin is natural or is derived from natural sources, it is synthetic; complicated chemical names also indicate a synthetic source.

Synthetic vitamins are valuable as therapeutic agents when extremely large doses of fast-acting vitamins are necessary. In this case they quickly and efficiently combat specific diseases which are caused by deficiency.

BASIC HEALTH DIET

The most recent research indicates that our past beliefs in regard to a high protein requirement are incorrect. Our daily intake of protein should be no higher than 30 per cent and should come from grains, nuts and seeds rather than from meat, poultry and dairy products. A high-animal-protein diet is now considered detrimental to health and may cause or contribute to many of our most common diseases. Proteins, although essential to life, can be harmful when consumed in excess; the metabolism of excess leaves toxic residues in the tissues and causes over-acidity. Emphasis should be on three basic foods: grains/nuts/seeds, vegetables and fruits; in addition we need adequate supplies of milk and other dairy products, vegetable oils and honey – and minimum amounts of meat, poultry and fish.

This is quite different from what most of us are accustomed to. At first the limitations on flesh foods may seem too difficult and too unrealistic, but in fact the main adjustment involved is to the main meal of the day, where smaller portions could lead to partial elimination. The proportions of nutrients have to be differently balanced, with much more use made of grains and vegetables. Try and take 50 per cent of the daily diet raw – this requires considerable re-thinking and effort. Natural therapists would like us to eat 80 per cent of our food raw – this proportion is insisted on for therapeutic régimes. Cooking can destroy much of the nutritional value; it also changes the biochemical structure of amino and fatty acids, making them only partially digestible.

The following rules should be observed for healthy eating:

Select only fresh wholesome food.

Eliminate sugar, refined grains and flours, and bread made with refined flour.

Eat as little fat as possible: vegetable oils are preferable, though small amounts of butter are permitted.

Take care, when cooking, that the nutrient value is not destroyed (see page 236).

Eat as much raw food as possible, at least 50 per cent of daily intake.

Coarse-ground grains, wholewheat flours and breads are ideal staple foods.

The best supplements to the basic diet are brewer's yeast, yogurt, honey, wheatgerm and kelp.

Eat only when hungry, even if it means missing a meal; nature has provided a built-in mechanism to tell you when you should eat or drink; food eaten without appetite does little good.

It is better to eat several small meals a day than two huge ones; this would help solve low-blood-sugar problems.

Try not to mix too many foods at the same meal, particularly raw foods; raw fruits and vegetables require different gastric juices from other foods, and are better eaten at different times.

DAILY GUIDE

On rising	Glass of water, plain or combined with the juice of a freshly squeezed citrus fruit – lemon, grapefruit, orange
	or
	a cup of herb tea, sweetened with honey – peppermint, camomile, rose hip or any favourite
Breakfast	Contrary to what most nutritionists say, this should be light as the stomach is not usually ready for much food, and a heavy breakfast uses up energy in digestion.
	fresh fruit in season (alone or as a salad) with yogurt
	or
	muesli (see page 280 for recipe) with yogurt
	or
	whole-grain cereal, such as rolled oats or bran
	slice of wholewheat toast, with a little butter and honey
	herb tea
Mid-morning	Fruit or vegetable juice
Lunch	Vegetable or fruit salad (oil and lemon dressing)
	or
	vegetable soup from greens, pods, seeds
	or
	cooked vegetables
	nuts, cheese
	wholewheat bread
Dinner	As lunch, but an egg, cheese, meat, poultry or fish dish (though preferably not every day) may be added

This may look like a skimpy menu, but there is a wide range of foods to choose from. See the recipes on pages 249–89 for ideas on how to present them – it is up to you what you do within this framework. It is good to drink as much water as possible; herb teas are preferable to regular tea and coffee; have alcohol and wine if you want to.

There is a cereal from Abe Waerland, one of the early pioneers of health through sensible eating, that provides top nutrition and energy, and is used by many clinics:

Waerland Kruska

(to serve four persons)

1 tablespoon whole wheat

1 tablespoon whole oats

1 tablespoon whole rye

1 tablespoon whole millet

1 tablespoon whole barley

2 tablespoons wheat bran

2 tablespoons raisins

Grind all the grains – a coffee-grinder works well – put in a pot with 1½ cups of water and add bran and raisins. Boil for 7 – 10 minutes, cover and allow to stand in a warm place for 2 hours. Serve with milk or stewed fruits. It can be made more quickly by boiling the water and pouring it over the grains, bran and raisins; allow to steep for ½ hour.

RAW JUICES

There is increasing emphasis on the value of raw vegetable and fruit juices within the concept of a basic daily health plan. They are used as supplements that provide concentrated forms of essential vitamins and minerals, enzymes and natural sugars. They can be used therapeutically to help specific diseases (see Part Two, The Power of Plants). For healthy people, they are recommended as between-meal fortifiers and as a preventive measure. Raw juices have a cleansing and detoxifying effect; they provide an alkaline surplus which is very important for balancing the acid–alkaline ratio in the blood and tissues – the over-acidity is the cause of many disorders. Juices purify the blood and the tissues, neutralize waste products and help build new cells. The following charts indicate the composition of the common fruits and vegetables; the figures should be taken as a general guide because amounts vary according to origin, freshness and climate. One to two glasses (about 1 pint or 6 dl.) of raw juices a day are of tremendous benefit to the system.

All raw juices are recommended, and which you take for general health is a matter of personal preference. Apple and the citrus fruits are the most popular of the sweet juices, while in the vegetable group, carrot is the most versatile; it goes well with other juices – celery, beet or cucumber, for example. The following is a green juice, rich in nutrients and valuable chlorophyll: put 2 cups of carrot juice in the blender and add any available greens, chopped (lettuce, kale, cabbage, turnip tops, spinach, parsley) and whisk until thoroughly blended.

COMPOSITION OF FRUIT JUICES
(mg. per 100 g.)

	Apple	Apricot	Grapefruit	Lemon	Orange	Papaya	Pineapple
Protein	0·2	0·6	0·5	0·7	0·8	0·6	0·5
Fat	trace	trace	trace	trace	trace	trace	trace
Carbohydrate	10	6·5	9	8	12·5	9	11·5
Carotene (for vitamin A)	0·04	1·5	0·02	—	0·05	1	0·05
Vitamin B-1	0·04	0·03	0·04	0·04	0·03	0·03	0·08
Vitamin B-2	0·03	0·05	0·02	trace	0·03	0·03	—
Vitamin B-3	0·1	0·5	0·2	0·2	0·2	0·2	0·1
Vitamin B-5	0·06	0·3	0·2	0·2	0·15	—	0·18
Vitamin B-6	0·04	—	0·06	0·06	0·03	—	—
Biotin (B complex)	0·3	—	0·2	—	0·8	—	—
Folic acid (B complex)	1	3	2	7	trace	40	4
Vitamin C	25	8	38	50	50	100	25
Vitamin E	0·7	—	—	—	0·3	—	0·1
Calcium	3	16	9	22	30	330	12
Chlorine	0·7	85·5	—	—	—	—	30
Copper	0·8	0·35	—	—	—	—	0·08
Iron	0·85	0·35	0·2	0·5	0·5	0·5	0·5
Magnesium	4	12	12	8	13	—	17
Manganese	0·04	0·01	—	—	—	—	—
Phosphorus	13	20	11	12	33	—	7·7
Potassium	100	340	163	123	195	—	245
Sodium	2	0·5	1	1	3	—	1·5
Sulphur	6	6	—	—	9	—	2·5
Zinc	0·01	0·08	—	—	9	—	2·5

COMPOSITION OF VEGETABLE JUICES
(mg. per 100 g.)

	Artichoke	Avocado	Beets	Brussels sprouts	Cabbage	Carrot	Celery	Cucumber	Green beans
Protein	3	1·2	1·3	3·5	33	1	0·9	0·6	0·8
Fat	trace	8·5	trace	trace	trace	trace	trace	trace	trace
Carbohydrate	15	2·5	6·5	4·5	3·4	45	1·3	1·8	1
Carotene (for vitamin A)	—	0·1	trace	—	1·5	6–12	—	—	0·5
Vitamin B-1	0·2	0·7	0·3	0·8	0·05	0·06	0·03	0·04	0·5
Vitamin B-2	0·01	0·15	0·05	0·2	0·05	0·06	0·03	0·04	0·1
Vitamin B-3	0·1	1	0·1	0·7	0·25	0·6	0·3	0·2	0·6
Vitamin B-5	—	—	0·13	0·4	0·18	0·25	0·4	0·3	0·1
Vitamin B-6	—	—	0·05	0·28	0·12	0·1	0·1	0·04	0·1
Biotin (B complex)	—	—	trace	0·4	0·1	0·6	0·1	—	1·2
Folic acid (B complex)	—	—	20	30	20	10	7	6	—
Vitamin C	8	18	6	87	53	8	9	8	10
Vitamin E	—	—	—	—	0·1	0·5	0·5	—	—
Calcium	50	15·2	25	29	45	28	43	30	25
Chlorine	85·6	6	61	35	23	72	183	25·6	60
Copper	0·1	0·2	0·08	0·05	0·06	0·1	trace	0·08	0·08
Iron	1	0·6	0·4	0·7	2·4	1·6	1·1	0·6	0·4
Magnesium	27	30	16	20	16	9·4	8·6	9	16
Manganese	—	0·08	0·08	0·1	0·06	0·01	0·01	0·06	0·28
Phosphorus	44	31	32·3	80	30	36	20	20	33
Potassium	330	400	300	515	260	315	245	150	320
Sodium	2·5	15	85	9·5	7	85	88	14	85
Sulphur	16·2	18·6	92	102	90	7	14·9	12	—
Zinc	—	—	0·3	0·37	0·14	0·12	0·07	0·1	0·3

Garlic	Horse-radish	Lettuce	Onion	Parsley	Potato	Spinach	Tomato	Turnip	Water-cress	
6·3	4·5	1	1	5·3	2·2	5·5	1	0·8	3	Protein
0·2	trace	trace	trace	trace	trace	trace	trace	trace	trace	Fat
30·8	11	1·9	5·4	trace	20	1·5	3	3·9	0·8	Carbohydrate
trace	—	1–3	—	8	trace	6	0·6	6·2	3	Carotene (for vitamin A)
0·25	0·07	0·07	0·03	0·15	0·12	0·12	0·06	0·03	0·1	Vitamin B-1
—	—	0·08	0·05	0·3	0·03	0·2	0·05	0·4	0·17	Vitamin B-2
0·5	—	0·3	0·2	1	1·3	0·7	0·6	0·5	0·6	Vitamin B-3
—	—	—	0·1	0·03	0·3	0·3	0·06	0·02	0·1	Vitamin B-5
—	—	—	0·1	0·2	0·2	0·1	0·1	0·1	—	Vitamin B-6
—	—	—	0·9	0·4	0·1	0·1	1·3	0·1	0·4	Biotin (B complex)
—	—	—	10	40	6	80	5	4	50	Folic acid (B complex)
15	81	15	10	150	20	60	20	25	60	Vitamin C
—	—	0·5	0·3	—	0·1	—	0·4	2·2	3	Vitamin E
29	120	26	22	330	8	483	13·5	59	325	Calcium
—	19	41	21	160	79	53	52	70	160	Chlorine
—	0·14	0·15	0·1	0·5	0·15	0·25	0·1	0·1	0·2	Copper
1·5	2·13	0·75	0·75	8	0·75	4·5	0·4	0·4	1·6	Iron
36	35·8	10	10	56	25	84·5	10	7	18	Magnesium
—	—	0·07	0·08	—	—	—	—	—	—	Manganese
202	70	30	33	134	41	95	22	29	54	Phosporus
530	560	208	140	1,100	570	470	300	240	315	Potassium
19	8	3·1	10	35	6·5	362	3	56	60	Sodium
—	215	12	52	—	35	64	11	21	130	Sulphur
—	—	0·25	0·11	—	—	—	—	—	—	Zinc

METABOLIC CLEANSING

There are ways to clean out the body, getting rid of the toxic matter and waste that accumulate and destroy. This is essential when illness is the result, but even a seemingly healthy person can benefit from a metabolic rest from time to time, going on special mono-diets or by juice fasting. On a curative or long-term basis it is essential that this is done under the supervision of a doctor or natural therapist; as a health routine, it can be undertaken without supervision. Because all these régimes drastically reduce food intake or eliminate it altogether, they result in weight loss; indeed, the treatment may be geared to that end. The health aim is to eliminate destructive elements, to renew metabolism and prepare the body for acceptance of a diet of wholesome food.

THE GRAPE DIET

This is well-known and used in many clinics; it helps the whole body and tends to restore health. Grapes are rich in natural sugar and contain certain acids and traces of mineral salts. Eat only grapes, on the average 4 lb. ($1 \cdot 8$ kg.) a day, including the skins and some of the pips – be sure to wash them thoroughly first. This can be continued for up to ten days on your own, much longer when under supervision. People suffering from a variety of disorders of the stomach, liver and bowels have reported much improvement. As well as cleansing the blood the treatment often clears the skin. It is a good way to lose weight.

THE MILK DIET

This eliminates fluids by stimulating the kidneys. For four days only, drink four glasses of milk diluted with $1\frac{3}{4}$ pints (1 l.) Vichy water daily. It helps those who suffer from water retention (which means that toxic matter is held in the body); it may also help those with heart trouble.

THE SCROTH DIET

This is an old European metabolic 'cure' that should only be carried out under supervision, as it lasts on average for three weeks and sometimes involves the application of cold-water body packs (see Environment, page

63). It is good for those who suffer from fluid retention or diseases of the joints, skin and liver. It is used by many natural therapists.

Diet A

Only small quantities of liquid are permitted.

Morning	An early morning enema; toasted wholewheat bread allowed during the morning in any amount
Mid-day	Up to 18 oz. (500 g.) cooked oatmeal or brown rice with prunes
From mid-afternoon to 7 p.m.	Up to 4½ fl. oz. (125 c.c.) fruit juice or warm wine
7 p.m.	Porridge made from unpolished rice, semolina or barley
Bedtime	Cold body pack, if necessary

Diet B

Large quantities of liquid are taken.

Until mid-day	Only toasted wholewheat bread
Mid-day	Up to 12 oz. (350 g.) cooked oatmeal with stewed apples
Mid-afternoon to bedtime	Up to 18 fl. oz. (500 c.c.) of herb tea, fruit juice or wine

Diet C

No liquids at all. Toasted wholewheat bread and dried prunes can be taken at intervals during the day. Thirst can be quenched by sucking on a few pieces of lemon. Sometimes a cold pack is applied in the evening.

The régime is as follows over a week: on days 1 and 4 take diet A; on days 3 and 6 take diet B; and on days 2, 5 and 7 take diet C. It is usual to continue for three weeks.

JUICE FASTING

This is the most effective and therapeutic body cleansing. Fasting is the oldest healing method, but with the emphasis on drug-orientated medicine it has been somewhat overlooked. The situation is now changing: scientific studies and clinical results both indicate the preventive, therapeutic and regenerative effects of fasting. The classical method was a water-only fast, but now authorities agree that juice fasting is far superior, as the alkali-forming fruit and vegetable juices accelerate the cleansing and healing process.

Advocates of fasting believe that to be effective a fast should last a minimum of a week, but not more than ten days without supervision. Under professional guidance, a fast can go on for months for special curative reasons and in cases of extreme obesity. Research shows that no harm is done, only good. Apart from health benefits, a fast usually results in an average loss in weight of 18 oz. (500 g.) per day after the first three days. After the third day the body starts to live on its own substance and any early hunger symptoms disappear,

The body will actually burn and digest its own tissues by the process of autolysis. Cells and tissues which are diseased, damaged, old or dead are the first to decompose – this process of getting rid of the unnecessary first is one of the more startling aspects of fasting. The essential tissues and vital organs are not touched or damaged. Because the old tissues are eliminated, the building of new healthy cells is speeded up. During this process, the eliminating organs – lungs, liver, kidneys and skin – are working hard getting rid of waste matter and toxins; this is evident in bad breath, dark urine, sweating and sometimes skin break-outs.

Fasting gives a rest to the digestive and protective organs. It helps stabilize nerves and stimulates the mind. The glandular and hormone network is also stimulated, while the vitamin and mineral balance is normalized. All this is helped considerably by the intake of juices.

The clinic with the most experience in fasting is that of Dr Otto Buchinger in Germany (see Health Spas, page 94). This is their general régime, which can be taken as a schedule for limited fasting at home.

Fasting Schedule

For two or three days before fasting prepare the body by eating nothing but raw vegetables and fruits; one meal a day of any fruit, the other of any vegetable; do not mix both at the same meal. Fasting should begin with a good bowel cleansing – at the Buchinger Clinic a dose of Glauber's salt is given on the morning of the first fast day: $1\frac{1}{2}$ oz. (40 g.) salts in $\frac{1}{4}$ pint (1·5 dl.) warm water; this is followed by a glass of fruit juice. The daily diet schedule is always the same, with an enema given every morning or on alternate days.

Upon rising	enema
9 a.m.	Cup of herb tea, warm not hot (choose from any; specially recommended are peppermint, camomile, rose hip, ginseng)
11 a.m.	Glass of fresh fruit juice, diluted 1:1 with water
1 p.m.	Glass of fresh vegetable juice or a cup of vegetable broth (see recipe below)
4 p.m.	Cup of herb tea
7 p.m.	Glass of fresh fruit or vegetable juice, diluted 1:1 with water
9 p.m.	Cup of vegetable broth

Plain warm water or mineral water can be drunk when thirsty. The total juice volume, however, together with the broth should be between $1\frac{1}{2}$ pints (9 dl.) and $1\frac{1}{2}$ quarts (18 dl.). The above plan is the juice guide only; the régime at the clinic also includes exercise, rest periods, therapeutic baths.

Vegetable Broth
This should be freshly made each day. It is a standard beverage at many biological clinics. It is a cleansing and alkalizing drink, supplying vitamins and minerals too.
2 large potatoes, unpeeled and chopped
1 cup carrots, unpeeled and sliced
1 cup celery including leaves, chopped
1 cup red beets, finely sliced
1 cup any other available vegetable – cabbage, turnips, spinach, zucchini

Put $1\frac{1}{2}$ quarts (18 dl.) water in a pan (not aluminium or copper). Slice the vegetables directly into the water so as not to expose them to the air. Cook slowly for 45 minutes; allow to stand for 15 minutes; strain.

During fasting, it is important to observe these rules:

No smoking or drinking.

Do not take even a morsel of any food, otherwise the gastric juices will start to work and the benefits of the fast will be lost.

Withdrawal of drugs is advisable; exceptions are usually digitalis for the heart, insulin in diabetes and cortisone in arthritis.

Vitamins should be discontinued, unless otherwise stated by the doctor.

Regular work can be continued.

Exercise is very helpful, particularly in the fresh air.

Do not lie around in bed, it could be harmful.

Daily baths are important to wash away toxins eliminated through the skin; the pores must be kept open.

It is advisable to take an enema every day or every other day; during a fast toxins and waste matter are mainly eliminated by way of the kidneys and bowels; natural bowel movements cease during a fast, so an enema is needed to help evacuate the waste. This can be done with an enema or douche bag with $1\frac{1}{2}$ pints (9 dl.) of water (add a few drops of fresh lemon juice). Try to retain the water for a short while, before letting it out.

BREAKING A FAST

This is as important as the fast itself, for the success of the time of abstinence will depend on the way you come out of it. The rule is to take it easy; do not overeat; do not rush back to old ways. Take it slowly and think; one reason for fasting was to prepare the body to adjust to a continuous healthy diet. It takes several days to return to normal.

First Day

Breakfast	Half an apple, herb tea
11 a.m.	Glass of fresh fruit juice
1 p.m.	Cup of vegetable broth, bowl of fresh vegetable soup

4 p.m.	Herb tea
7 p.m.	Glass of fresh fruit juice
9 p.m.	Cup of vegetable broth

Second Day

Breakfast	Dish of soaked prunes, herb tea
11 a.m.	Glass of fresh fruit juice
1 p.m.	Small bowl of vegetable salad
4 p.m.	One apple
7 p.m.	Bowl of vegetable soup
9 p.m.	Cup of vegetable broth

Third Day

Breakfast	Soaked prunes, yogurt, a few ground nuts, herb tea
11 a.m.	One apple
1 p.m.	Larger portion of vegetable salad baked potato cup of vegetable broth
4 p.m.	One apple
7 p.m.	Bowl of vegetable soup slice of wholewheat bread with butter slice of cheese
9 p.m.	Cup of vegetable broth

On the fourth day a normal diet can commence, slowly bringing in the full range of wholesome foods according to the Basic Health Diet, pages 13–16. Therapeutic fasting can be undertaken again after an interval of six weeks.

VEGETARIANISM

This is a diet that eliminates flesh food such as meat, fish and fowl; milk, cheese, butter, cream and eggs are taken as well as vegetables, fruits, grains, and nuts; honey is used for sweetening. Vegetarians were once considered eccentrics, but modern research reveals that there are many benefits from a meatless diet. It is quite possible to get all the necessary vitamins and minerals without eating flesh foods and children mature in a healthy way on a vegetarian diet.

Protein is essential in any diet and vegetarians must be particularly careful to include an adequate amount in their daily menu. Actually, as vegetarians are so conscious of their nutrients they usually take just the right amount of protein; normal western nutrition veers towards an excess, which leads to the onset of degenerative diseases. The awareness of the specific value of foods leads to greater awareness of other health patterns; exercise, particularly breathing and yoga disciplines, is often taken up.

VEGAN DIET

Vegans live solely on the products of plants, avoiding all animal produce: meat, fish, fowl, eggs, milk and its derivatives, and honey. It is usually adopted for ethical, ecological or health reasons.

This diet requires constant attention to nutrients, but it is quite possible to live healthily on it. The only problem is the deficiency of vitamin B–12, and it is advisable to take tablet supplements. The general health of vegans is good; they are inclined to weigh less and, because there is no intake of animal fats at all, cholesterol levels are low, which decreases the chance of circulatory and heart troubles.

It is best to change gradually from an omnivorous diet to a vegan or vegetarian one, experimenting with plant sources and gradually adjusting the body to the new eating plan.

MACROBIOTIC FOOD

Many people are under the impression that this is a very restricted diet; in fact it follows the general rules of healthy eating, with more emphasis on grains, which should comprise 50 per cent of the diet. It allows fish and fowl as secondary foods, but they have to be combined with grains and vegetables in a meal.

The principle of *yin* and *yang* – the theory of complementary opposites – governs the selection of food in the macrobiotic diet. This corresponds more or less to acidity and alkalinity; acid foods are rich in potassium, alkaline in sodium. *Yin* also represents the passive principle and *yin* foods include fruits, drinks, foods of sweet, sour or hot flavour, summer-maturing foods and those of purple, blue or green colour. *Yang* is masculine; *yang* foods include foods of animal origin, cereals and some vegetables; they are usually compact and hard and red, yellow or orange in colour; they are salty or bitter to taste and usually mature in the autumn or winter.

The perfect balance is considered 5:1 – five parts *yin* (potassium) to one part *yang* (sodium). This perfect balance is found in only one food, brown rice. However, it is definitely not advisable to eat only one food of any type and brown rice is no exception. A nutritious diet includes a wide variety of foods and most macrobiotics eat many combinations of foods to achieve the 5:1 ratio. Other grains come near to the ideal, so wholewheat, rye, barley, oats, millet, buckwheat and maize together with brown rice are the principal foods. Vegetables and pulses supplement the grains; fish and poultry are eaten occasionally and wild plants and seaweeds when available. Soy-bean products are important – particularly *miso* and *tamari*, a purée and a liquid soy sauce made by natural lactic fermentation of soy beans over eighteen months or more; they are a rich source of amino acids and give great flavour to the grain foods. The recommended tea is *mu* tea, a compound of fifteen roots and herbs, including ginseng. Drinks – even tea and water – are kept to a minimum.

No processed foods are used, nor is sugar or any refined carbohydrates; potatoes, tomatoes and eggplant are taken, but with caution. The emphasis is on food in its most natural form, with no processing beyond quick and minimum cooking. Foods of local origin are preferred, as macrobiotics believe there is an affinity between people of a region and the foods that grow there.

A ten-day rice diet is sometimes used as a cleansing routine for the digestive system; nothing but brown rice is eaten for this period. An extended brown-rice diet can sometimes be harmful, despite the fact that macrobiotic fans say it is possible to exist on this grain alone. Keep track of how the body is reacting and adjust your diet accordingly.

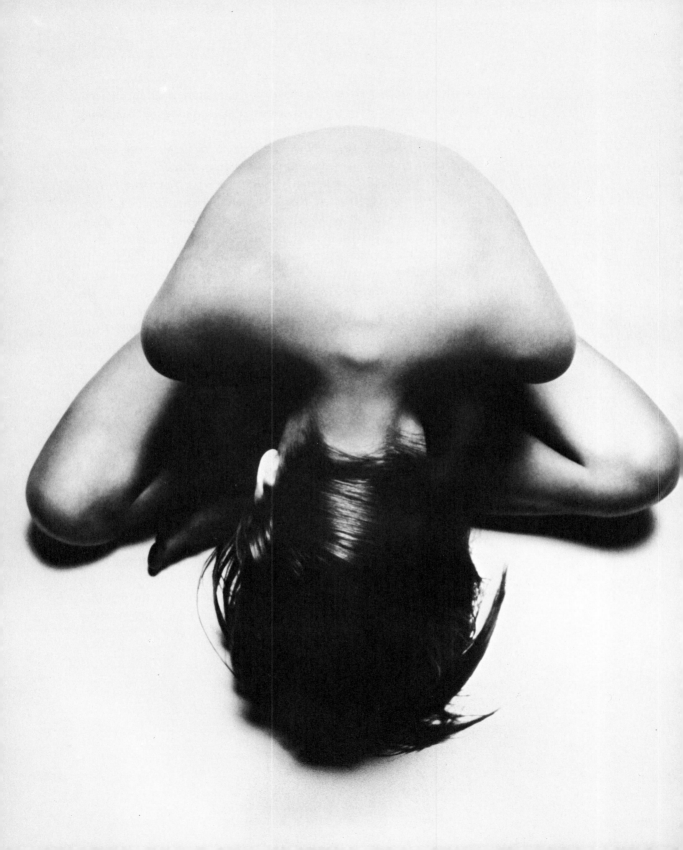

2

MOVEMENT

Do you really know your body? How it looks, how it feels, how it is at rest or in action? Body consciousness is the prime motivation of improvement. To be able to see, feel, sense and assess what is wrong is the first step to doing something about it. We all misuse our bodies to some degree, causing physical and organic disturbances. Yet by means of movement, we can re-shape the body within its skeletal limits, we can improve health, provide energy, stimulate metabolic functions, relieve tension, stabilize emotions and sharpen the mind. All this through constructive body use.

Posture is fundamental. Most of us are off-balance, holding the body in unnatural positions – putting more weight on one side than the other, twisting to left or right, allowing one shoulder to drop, keeping the head tilted. Whatever initially causes wrong posture, in time it becomes a habit. Poor posture leads to faulty coordination and movement, to wrong use of muscles, to incorrect breathing and, invariably, to tension. Its effect on general health is far-reaching. Re-education is of great importance for anyone who has forgotten the correct way to stand, sit, walk or relax. A pioneer in this field was Matthias Alexander who, after re-educating his own body through self-observance and diligent correction, developed a system now known as the Alexander Technique. It is a method of showing people how they are misusing their bodies and how to correct bad habits. Teachers explain and convey information through manual adjustment and at the same time a new mental process is taught to overcome the earlier automatic responses. It is difficult to readjust on both physical and mental levels; it requires discipline and concentration. There is no instant reversal but with intense mental application for short periods at a time, new posture habits will slowly build up and eventually become automatic.

An instructor is a great help, because few people can change stance and automatic movement without objective opinion and guidance. For self-assessment, here are some general rules on correct alignment and body use.

POSTURE

The spine is not straight and should not be straightened. It is a series of curves, the core of the body, and only the bones in the upper part depart from the central line. The curved ribs are joined to the twelve spinal bones of the upper back, so any over-straight or slumped position will hamper rib movements and consequently affect breathing. If the upper part of the back is held correctly, the shoulders will fall into place. The bones of the lower back are larger and strong; the curve should be just right – not too hollow otherwise the stomach will stick out, not too straight or back-aches result. One common mistake is to bend the back when stooping or lifting – you should bend the pelvis and knee joints, with the back still held in alignment. Check your posture in a full-length mirror, check for even balancing of weight, check the horizontal as well as vertical positions. Verbally and mentally direct the body into a correct position; think about lengthening and widening the back, think about releasing the neck and holding the head straight and untilted. Let the mind make the body work.

STANDING

Feet should be in line and a little apart, toes pointing slightly out. Body weight should be spread evenly over the whole surface of both feet. Relax the feet and uncurl the toes – do not grip the floor with them. Legs should be straight but not braced backwards. Straighten the spine by imagining there is a thread running through it which is being pulled up tautly from above your head; in this way the stretching is at the back of the neck, which holds the head in proper alignment and prevents rigidness at the base of the spine. Arms should hang loosely at the sides.

SITTING

Slumping must be avoided; also uneven lounging with the weight pushed to one side. The spine should be straight without being stretched, shoulders neither braced nor drooping. Feet firmly on the floor, slightly apart, but free of tension. The buttocks support the body; avoid the inclination to lean on arms and elbows – hands should be on thighs.

WALKING

The same upright posture as in standing should be maintained with conscious balancing of the head, neck muscles and spine. The head should be held high, chin neither tucked in nor jutting out. The body should be upright but not braced, nor should the pelvis be thrust too far forward as this upsets the balance. Movement should come from the thighs, not the hips, though the hips remain relaxed and not held in a rigid position. Be aware of the flexibility of feet and ankles during walking.

YOGA

One of the east's oldest self-improvement concepts, yoga is still the best body discipline. It consists of breathing exercises, postures and movements. But it goes deeper than that, for yoga is also a mind process, a way to self-awareness and self-realization. In the west we have adopted it primarily as a way of therapeutic exercise; through it you can achieve complete relaxation of mind and body. You can learn to breathe properly, to bring energy to mental and physical processes, to become more flexible and supple. Its postures and principles are also health-giving in that they relieve tension and stimulate the circulatory, endocrine and nervous systems. Last, though not least, yoga can improve the shape, grace and beauty of a body.

Always begin any yoga session by relaxing completely for a few minutes. The next step is learning to breathe, to appreciate the value and power of *prana* (air); then you are ready to limber up with a few simple movements before tackling the postures. It is imperative to take it slowly; never overstrain; learn the disciplines step by step. Concentration is the key; it is more significant than control and achievement, and is the only way to achieve either.

The basic pose for yoga is the Lotus position. Sit on the ground with legs straight in front. Bend your right leg and with your hands lift the right foot, placing it, sole upwards, against the left groin. Now take hold of the other foot, bending the knee, and place it in the right groin. This takes considerable practice. However, it is not essential to be in this position either for breathing or for meditative sessions; the simple cross-legged position will do instead.

A sequence of routines is illustrated and explained on the following pages. Yoga should be performed in an airy room on the hard floor with a rug or mat for protection. Don't wear restrictive clothing – no clothes, or an easy garment of natural fibre, is best.

BREATHING

In the beginning is breath; this is the prime principle of yoga. Prana *is the word for breath, but it means not only air, but all of life; it is vitality, energy, power, strength; it is spirit and soul too. Yogis believe that if you can control and use breath properly, its energy can positively influence body and mind. Good respiration brings back mobility of the lungs and the abdomen; it is learning to breathe with the whole, instead of with only part, of the lungs. The posture in which you study breathing is significant and the kind of thoughts that accompany the breath are important. Here is a series of breathing techniques to teach you the art of* pranayama. *Always breathe in and out through the nose, using these patterns for five minutes at a time at intervals during the day – in total about half an hour – by an open window.*

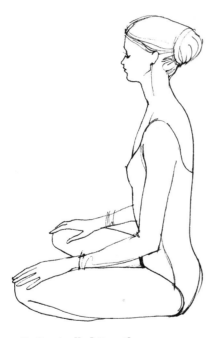

1. Controlled Breath

Sit down in the most comfortable pose, a simple crossed-legs or a Lotus position, where the thighs form a firm base; rest the hands on the knees, spine straight, head high and balanced. Close the eyes for concentration and do the following breathing patterns.

For energy: Exhale deeply; take a deep breath from the stomach and release air by forcefully jerking the abdomen, exhaling through the nose; do not let go of all the air at once – pause for a second; jerk again to expel more air, pause; release until lungs are empty. Then take in a long slow breath through the nose, hold it to the count of five and slowly exhale. Repeat this sequence five times.

For power: Exhale deeply; breathe in slowly, thinking of air's life-giving energy, its power to heal. Hold to the count of seven and release slowly, visualizing that you have sent that power to a particular part of the body. Repeat five times.

For mastery: Exhale deeply; now breathe in until you feel the need to breathe out, but don't; instead take in another small breath, hold for a second and slowly exhale until you think all air has been expelled, hold for a second, push out just a little more. The rhythm is: in, hold, in again; out, hold, out again. Repeat five times.

2. Abdominal Breath

Lie on the floor with a pillow under the head, knees bent and touching, feet slightly apart. Be sure the spine is relaxed and in a straight line; yogis regard this important in order to allow the free flow of energy and thoughts. Place your hands over your stomach. Slowly breathe out and at the same time gently press hands up under your ribs; this will help push the air from the bottom of your lungs. Breathe in deeply and slowly, returning the hands to relaxed pressure on the stomach; as you are breathing in try to push the hands up with your stomach, but don't lift the body off the ground; push the hands up to the ribs and exhale. Relax hands and breathe in. Continue the rhythm for two minutes. During inhalation the stomach should rise as high as possible; it is not your ribs that move, it is the abdomen. This technique requires great concentration.

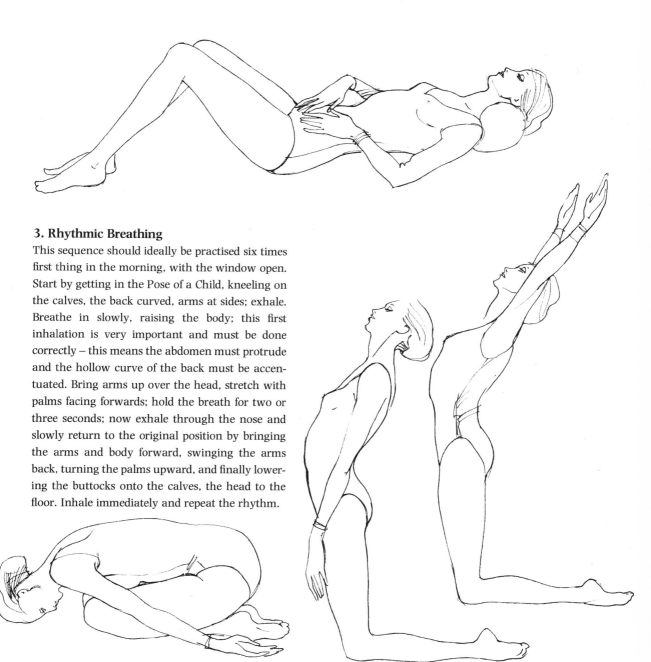

3. Rhythmic Breathing

This sequence should ideally be practised six times first thing in the morning, with the window open. Start by getting in the Pose of a Child, kneeling on the calves, the back curved, arms at sides; exhale. Breathe in slowly, raising the body; this first inhalation is very important and must be done correctly – this means the abdomen must protrude and the hollow curve of the back must be accentuated. Bring arms up over the head, stretch with palms facing forwards; hold the breath for two or three seconds; now exhale through the nose and slowly return to the original position by bringing the arms and body forward, swinging the arms back, turning the palms upward, and finally lowering the buttocks onto the calves, the head to the floor. Inhale immediately and repeat the rhythm.

LIMBERING-UP

This group of movements is designed to bring greater flexibility to the body in preparation for the more demanding postures of yoga. In themselves, however, they offer a basic routine for daily body activity as they strengthen muscles which are usually neglected, increase circulation and energize the system. They should be done, not as physical jerks, but as slow controlled patterns with good breathing technique. Before starting, relax the body by shaking it, first the hands and arms, then the feet and legs.

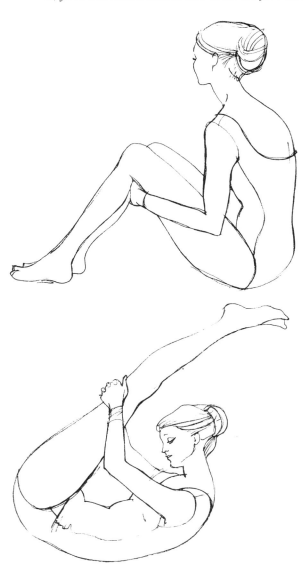

1. Spinal Roll

Sit on the floor, knees up and hands clasped underneath them; the back should be slightly curved. Slowly roll backwards, straightening the legs as they go over the head; roll forwards to the sitting position, bending the knees as you return to the original position. Go rhythmically back and forth ten times. Relax by lying flat on the back, breathing calmly for a minute or two. The exercise is good for the spine, helping to keep it supple.

2. Knee Stretch (Illustration opposite)

First lie flat on the floor, then gently bend one knee, bringing it up as far as possible over the chest towards the chin, at the same time bringing the head forward to meet the knee. Hold to the count of three; return slowly. Do this three times and then repeat with the other leg. With practice, increase the length of time the knee is held in position and the number of times the exercise is repeated. Take it slowly, never strain; pull gently at first. This stretching affects the lower spinal area and the front and back of the legs.

3. Knees Bend (Illustration opposite)

An important exercise but not as simple as it sounds or looks. At first it is difficult to balance the body while keeping the bottom tucked under and the

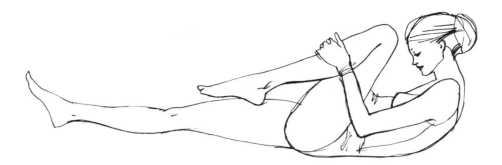

back straight. Start by squatting, keeping your feet more or less flat on the ground and bending forward, arms hanging in front for balance. Hold to the count of five; put your hands on your knees and push the body to an upright position. Do this three or four times before attempting the proper knees bend.

Stand straight, raise the toes and slowly lower the spine, bending the knees until you are sitting on your heels. Hands should be kept in a praying position in front of the body during the entire movement. Stay crouched to the count of five; slowly return to standing, lower heels. Repeat five times at first, working up to as many as possible without strain. This movement stretches the leg and back muscles and firms the thighs; it also helps develop control and balance. Breathe in as you go on tiptoe, out as you bend.

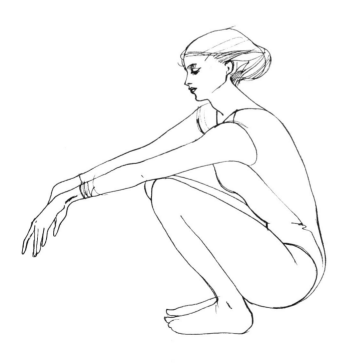

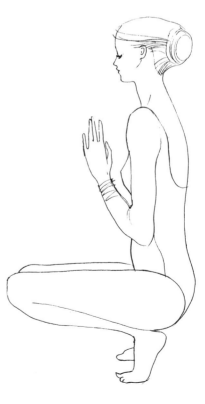

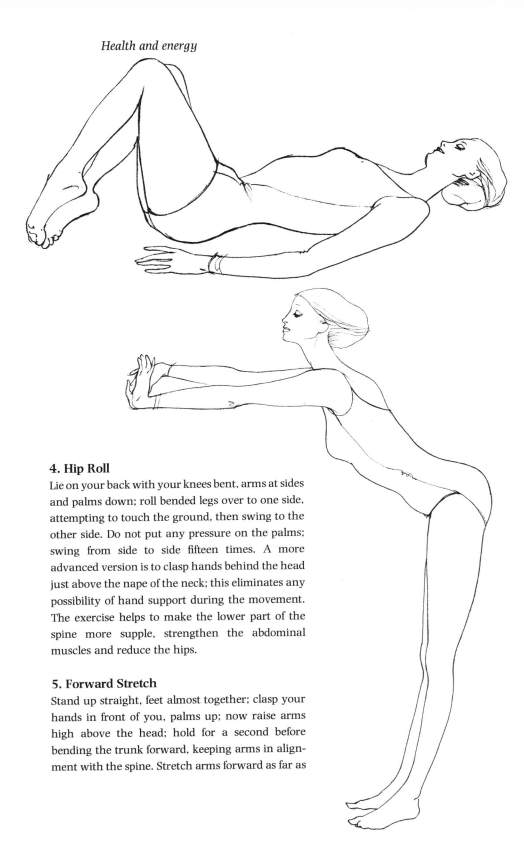

4. Hip Roll

Lie on your back with your knees bent, arms at sides and palms down; roll bended legs over to one side, attempting to touch the ground, then swing to the other side. Do not put any pressure on the palms; swing from side to side fifteen times. A more advanced version is to clasp hands behind the head just above the nape of the neck; this eliminates any possibility of hand support during the movement. The exercise helps to make the lower part of the spine more supple, strengthen the abdominal muscles and reduce the hips.

5. Forward Stretch

Stand up straight, feet almost together; clasp your hands in front of you, palms up; now raise arms high above the head; hold for a second before bending the trunk forward, keeping arms in alignment with the spine. Stretch arms forward as far as

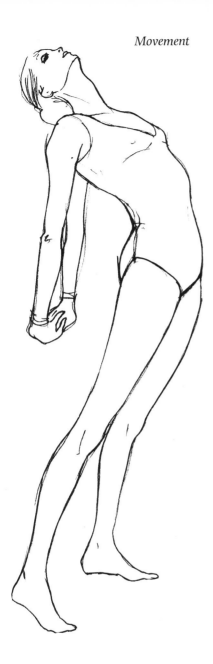

6. Backward Stretch

From an upright standing position, bring the arms back and interlace the fingers; raise the arms as high as possible, stretching outwards, and at the same time slowly bend backwards, arching the back but keeping the knees straight; hold to the count of five. Now gently bend forward, bringing your arms up over the back; arms and legs must be kept straight; bend forward as far as possible, aiming to touch your knees with your head; hold to the count of ten. Repeat three times. This helps flexibility and also chest expansion, facilitating correct breathing.

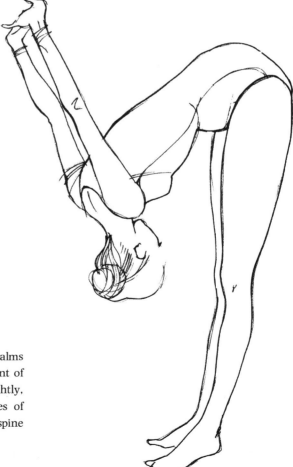

possible, hold to the count of five; now turn palms outwards, push and stretch, hold to the count of five; now push, stretch and lift the arms slightly, hold to the count of five. Repeat the series of movements three times; they are good for the spine and for stimulating the nervous system.

A RHYTHMIC SEQUENCE

This is a series of coordinated movement patterns, for those with limited time, based on yoga principles and poses. It is a stimulating way to start the day, but it can also act as a quick refresher course after working. Try to do the limbering-up movements first, then as many rounds of the sequence as possible – at least five minutes. Remember to take it slowly and smoothly, breathing properly and controlling the body through concentration and mind direction.

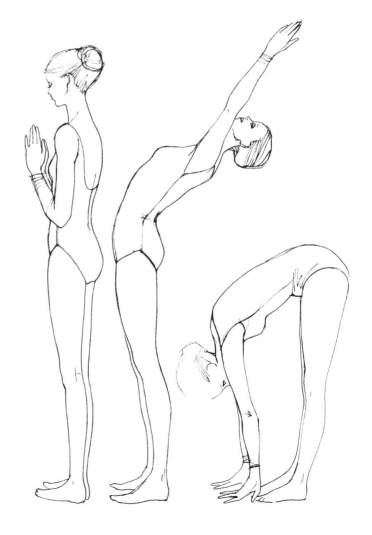

1. Stand straight with the feet to-gether, arms bent against the body and hands in a prayer position; take deep regulated breaths, exhaling slowly; direct the mind to body action and control. This establishes a state of relaxation and concentration.

2. Inhaling deeply, lift the arms over the head, moving the hands apart; stretch upwards and at the same time slightly arch the back. This flexes the spinal cord, exercises the arms and stretches the abdominal muscles.

3. Exhale slowly, bringing the arms down to the floor in front of the feet and gently bending the back; do not force this movement; go down only as far as is comfortable – it is not nec-essary to touch the floor; hold to the count of three. This helps to control and reduce the abdomen, provides more flexibility for the spine and tones the thigh and leg muscles.

4. Using the hands to support the body, bring the right leg back, stretch-ing to push as far back as possible, at the same time bending the left knee. Try to keep the back in a straight line,

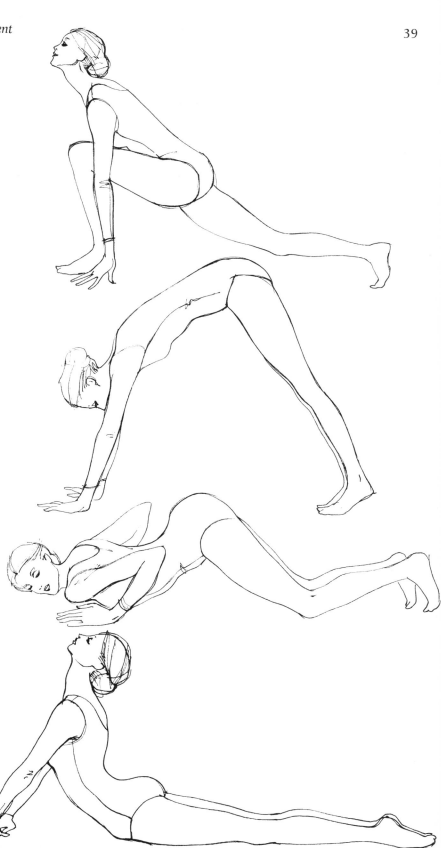

but stretch the neck so the head is tilted as if to catch the rays of the sun. Inhale to the count of three, relax. This stretches the spine and strengthens the leg muscles.

5. Put the palms flat on the floor and, supporting the body with the arms, bring back the left leg into exact alignment with the right; feet should be kept flat on the floor if possible; exhale when the position is reached and hold to the count of three. This stretches and stimulates the muscles of the arms and legs.

6. Inhale deeply, lowering the body to the floor by bending the arms and knees, but trying to keep the hips and abdomen raised; exhale and relax. This aids the nerves and muscles of the arms, shoulders and chest; it also helps to control the abdomen.

7. Lower the abdomen and hips and straighten the legs; inhale; using the hands as a support, raise the torso from the floor, arching the back and stretching the neck; hold to the count of three; exhale while slowly lowering body to the floor; relax. This limbers the spine and helps arm, shoulder, chest and neck muscles.

This sequence can be repeated in two ways – either return to the first position and repeat the series, or slowly return to the starting pose by reversing the sequence, going from posture seven to six, then forming the triangle, the plunge position, the touch-toes stretch and finally standing straight. The reverse movement is more difficult, requiring extra concentration and control.

YOGA POSTURES

Known as asanas, *they are calculated to have an effect on various functions and organs of the body. A minimum of motion is involved and everything is done at slow tempo, without strain. Always start and finish each posture with a few moments of complete relaxation. Asanas are performed in conjunction with deep rhythmic breathing and complete concentration; forget problems and all distractions. Control of consciousness is the ultimate aim and only if the mind gives undivided attention to what the body is doing will maximum influence be exerted on every muscle, nerve and cell. A certain amount of effort and motion are necessary to obtain them. At first you may only be able to master two or three, but that is not important. What counts is the daily routine of attempting to unite a mental, physical and spiritual experience. Do not dissipate energies; it is better to practice a single posture for a while, perfecting it before attempting another. Westerners find at first that limbs and joints ache. This is natural, but with time stiff muscles will limber up; any aching parts should be stretched briefly and gently massaged before moving on to the next position. This selection of postures is chosen for its suitability for beginners and because together it provides an all-round toning, shaping and health-giving programme. Rest briefly after each* asana, *and alternate the more invigorating ones with the relatively restful. Begin exercises with a few minutes of deep relaxation, followed by the breathing routines; limbering-up movements can be done if you like. Set aside a fixed time every day; try to do yoga* asanas *for twenty minutes daily; in the morning is best, before eating.*

The Plough

Lie flat on your back, legs outstretched, knees straight, arms by the side of the body, palms down. Lift the legs, keeping them straight, first to an angle of thirty degrees; pause for the count of three; continue upwards another thirty degrees, pause for the count of three; raise legs further to the vertical position, hold to the count of five; then slowly swing the legs over the head aiming to touch the floor with your toes. Your hands should remain flat on the floor, arms straight, knees straight. Slide the toes further away from the head. Hold this pose to the count of ten; reverse movements to starting position; relax. Breathing should be deep and regular throughout the *asana*. It is practically impossible to touch the floor with the toes at first – knees are inclined to bend, hands lift off the floor. If this is done slowly and perfectly, one performance is enough. It stretches the spine and abdominal muscles and helps circulation and endocrine actions.

The Pose of a Child

Start from a kneeling position with both the knees and feet together, arms at the sides. Slowly bend over to curve into a relaxed position, trying to bring the head down to the ground and as close to the knees as possible; arms follow the line of the legs. Hold to the count of ten; work up to holding for one or two minutes. This is a restful *asana*, a constructive way of relaxing the body after a strenuous movement; it also flexes the spine, aids abdominal muscles and helps to balance the nervous system.

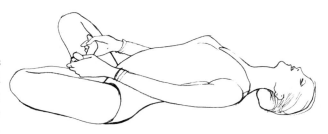

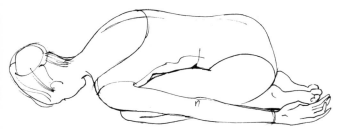

The Fish

The start is the Lotus pose (see page 31). Legs crossed, spine stretched, head balanced, hands on knees. Slowly lean backwards, using the elbows and arms for balance; concentrate and control muscles for a smooth backward gesture until the body forms an arc and your head is resting on the floor. Adjust for comfort. Now lift the hands from the knees and grasp the toes; stretch the arms, stretch the spine and counterbalance the forces of both. Hold to the count of five on first attempt, then ten, finally for a minute. This movement is good for general muscle toning but especially those in the base of the spine, the pelvis and the sacral region. Neck muscles are stimulated, helping tension; also helps respiratory troubles.

The Cat Stretch

Kneel down, with feet together and knees a little apart; buttocks should be resting on the ankles, back straight and arms at the side. Raise the arms over the head and at the same time bend over the torso bringing the head to the knees, the arms stretched out in front. Now aim to push as far forward as possible, sliding the hands on the floor and pulling the head away from the knees. The stretch starts from the hips. When in the extended position hold to the count of five; now roll to the right very slowly so that the right shoulder touches the floor, but keep the stretch extension, hold to the count of five. Roll to the other side, stretch, hold to the count of five. This posture flexes the spine, controls abdominal muscles, tones muscles in the arms and shoulders; it is said to relieve sciatica pains.

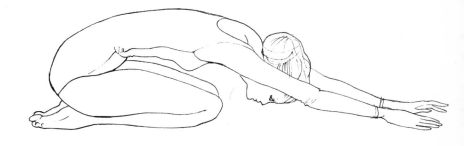

The Grip

This is often called the Head of a Cow. Kneel, with the buttocks resting on the heels, toes together, knees just slightly apart, back straight, arms hanging at sides. Bend the left arm behind the back, hand resting between shoulder blades with the palm facing outwards. Raise the right arm over the head, slowly bend backwards behind the neck to clasp the left hand; try to interlace fingers and pull gently in opposite directions; when final extension is reached hold to the count of five. Relax. Repeat with alternative arm movements. Calm concentration should coincide with this pose. The upper arm muscles are toned, the back is put into posture and conditioned to more flexibility.

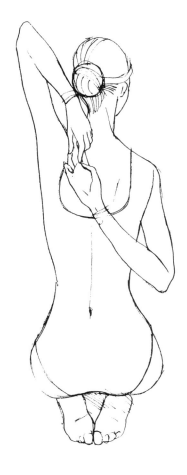

The Cobra

Lie on the stomach, face down with forehead touching the floor, but with arms bent so that the elbows are raised and the palms of the hands are flat on the floor just under the shoulders. The legs must be stretched straight, toes pointed, no bend in the knees; during the entire movement the knees must not be allowed to relax or bend in any way. Now slowly raise the head as high as possible, pushing the chin forward; the chest and torso need to be lifted off the ground as high as possible; the hands and arms give support, while the back takes most of the strain. It is only the front part of the torso that is raised, from the navel back to the toes everything should be on the floor and held straight. When you are finally upright, retain the posture for as long as possible without feeling strain; first do it to the count of three, then five, then ten, then hold for a full minute – this will take a lot of practice. Slowly return to the supine position; relax. The ideal is to not only be able to hold the position for a minute, but to do so with only fingertip support. At this point it only needs to be performed once a day. This movement is one of the best for spine suppleness and flexibility; it also firms the abdominal muscles and stimulates the kidney, liver and pancreas

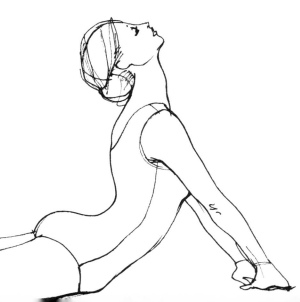

The Twist

First, sit on the floor with legs outstretched, hands at sides, palms on the floor; bend the right leg under the left thigh. Draw up the left leg, bending the knee until thigh and knee are resting against the abdomen and chest; lift the left foot over the right thigh and place the sole flat on the floor; the right hand should grasp the toes of the left foot but if this is difficult place it on the right knee (as in illustration). Keeping the palm of the left hand firmly on the floor, twist the torso to the left and hold this position for the length of three yoga breaths. Relax.

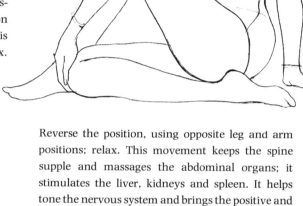

Reverse the position, using opposite leg and arm positions; relax. This movement keeps the spine supple and massages the abdominal organs; it stimulates the liver, kidneys and spleen. It helps tone the nervous system and brings the positive and negative forces of energy in the body to equilibrium.

Shoulder Stand

Start by lying flat on your back, legs outstretched, arms parallel to the body, palms down. Raise the legs slowly, keeping the knees straight and close together, toes pointing. Continue until legs are about a third of the way to a vertical position; pause briefly. Elevate the legs until vertical, stretch them, pause. Then pressing hands and elbows on the floor, also lift the torso, hips, back, stomach and chest, finally sliding your hands under the small of the back to help balance the trunk. Hold this posture for a few moments; slowly return to the original horizontal position. In time you should be able to hold the legs vertical for several minutes, without feeling any strain. This reverses the flow of blood which stimulates the endocrine system in general and particularly, it is believed, the thyroid. Muscles of the legs, thighs, hips, abdomen, shoulders, spine, neck and arms are all stretched.

T'AI-C'HI CHUAN

This is the Chinese equivalent of yoga. It is a form of moving meditation developed centuries ago, based on the movements of animals and many traditional fighting gestures. The heart of the Chinese concept is *ch'i*, which means air, with connotations of energy, spirit, power; it is the equivalent of the yoga *prana* and the western life force. The movements of *t'ai chi* illustrate the constant interplay between *yin* and *yang*, the passive and active forces. The mind is the focal point, air the catalyst and the body the medium. It encourages relaxation and mental peace; the effects are said to be both psychological and physiological.

The exercise pattern consists of a series of slow dance-like steps and gestures of the entire body. Particular attention is given to gravity and balance, to centering and to exactness of movement. There are no separate postures as such; the end of one movement becomes the beginning of the next. The weight of the body shifts continuously from one foot to the other and the movements are performed in circles, arcs and spirals. The body has to move as a unit.

There is no easy way to learn *t'ai chi* and it is very difficult to do it on one's own even with specific illustrated instructions. There are 108 basic forms that have to be learned, starting with coordination of mind and body and progressing to memorizing movements of limbs and eyes, then the relationship between movement and breathing and finally the balance between *yin* and *yang*. The Chinese say that one must practise for at least ten years before becoming a master. A trained instructor is necessary, and unfortunately there are not many available at the moment; the situation is improving, however, as this particular mind-and-matter movement is becoming more popular.

AEROBICS

These are natural body activities, such as walking, jogging, swimming, cycling, skipping (in other words non-competitive sports) that usually take place out of doors and involve increased intake of oxygen. This means they condition your heart, increasing cardiovascular capacity by stepping up the oxygen flow and utilization. It has been claimed that such programmes lessen the chance of prematurely developing coronary disease or related vascular ailments, as well as giving increased physical and mental alertness.

While specific callisthenic programmes aim to tone muscles and consequently trim the body, they do not usually raise your heart rate high enough to make a significant difference. What happens when you exercise aerobically is that your heart rate is pushed up to between 70 and 85 per cent of its maximum capacity. When done regularly this strengthens and enlarges the cardiac-pulmonary systems. The ultimate objective is to lower your resting heart rate and increase its stroke volume so that more blood reaches more tissues. In other words, aerobic training can increase your heart's efficiency, giving it built-in protection against strain during activity.

Needless to say, it is not advisable to rush into frenzied aerobic activity if you have been sedentary for years. A check with a doctor is advisable before any routine is undertaken.

Each of the following is comparable to the others in its aerobic training effect – any one of them, done two or three times a week, should give you all the exercise you need:

running two miles in less than twenty minutes;

swimming six hundred yards in less than fifteen minutes;

cycling five miles in less than twenty minutes;

stationary running for a total of twelve and a half minutes.

Checking your heart rate is a sensible precaution. Find a pulse point you can feel easily – the easiest to locate and record is the radial pulse located on the inside of the wrist, just below the hand on the thumb side. Use third and fourth fingers, firmly, but without applying pressure. Count pulse beat for exactly fifteen seconds and multiply by four to get the number of heart beats a minute. Now compare with the chart below.

Age	Threshold for training (70 per cent of maximum predicted beats a minute)	Limit not to be exceeded for peaks (85 per cent of maximum predicted beats a minute)	Maximum predicted beats a minute
20–24	140	170	200
25–9	140	170	200
30–34	136	165	194

Age	Threshold for training (70 per cent of maximum predicted beats a minute)	Limit not to be exceeded for peaks (85 per cent of maximum predicted beats a minute)	Maximum predicted beats a minute
35–9	132	160	188
40–44	128	155	182
45–9	124	150	176
50–54	119	145*	171
55–9	115	140*	165
60–64	111	135*	159

*Limitations for people over fifty must be rigidly followed.
A 130 limit for people over sixty is less than 85 per cent, but preferable.

A good home régime involves jogging and walking in place, gradually building up to an optimum performance. Use the chart and heart-rate figures to determine the intensity of the work-out you are getting. After one and a half to two minutes of exercising, take your pulse and check whether you are working too hard, or not hard enough. The precise timing of exercise and the effort exerted to reach the 70 per cent level will vary with each person. The speed at which you run and the height to which you raise your knees will also affect your heart rate. An initial trial-and-error period is necessary to establish your level. It is not necessary, nor advisable at first, to make it a daily routine; the suggested schedule is three days of exercise followed by one day of rest, then two days of exercise followed by one day of rest. Over the weeks you can build up to a more intensive level and finally make it a daily routine.

Weeks 1 and 2:   run two minutes (at least 70 per cent maximum heart rate)
walk in place one minute
run two minutes (at 70 per cent)
walk in place one minute
six minutes in all

Weeks 3 to 6:   run three minutes (at 70 per cent)
walk in place one minute
run three minutes (at 70 per cent)

walk in place one minute
eight minutes in all

Weeks 7 and 8:   run two minutes (at 70 per cent)
run one minute (at 85 per cent)
run one minute (at 70 per cent)
walk in place one minute
run three minutes (at 70 per cent)
walk in place one minute
nine minutes in all

From week 9:   run two minutes (at 70 per cent)
run one minute (at 85 per cent)
run one minute (at 70 per cent)
walk in place one minute
repeat the entire cycle three times: fifteen minutes in all

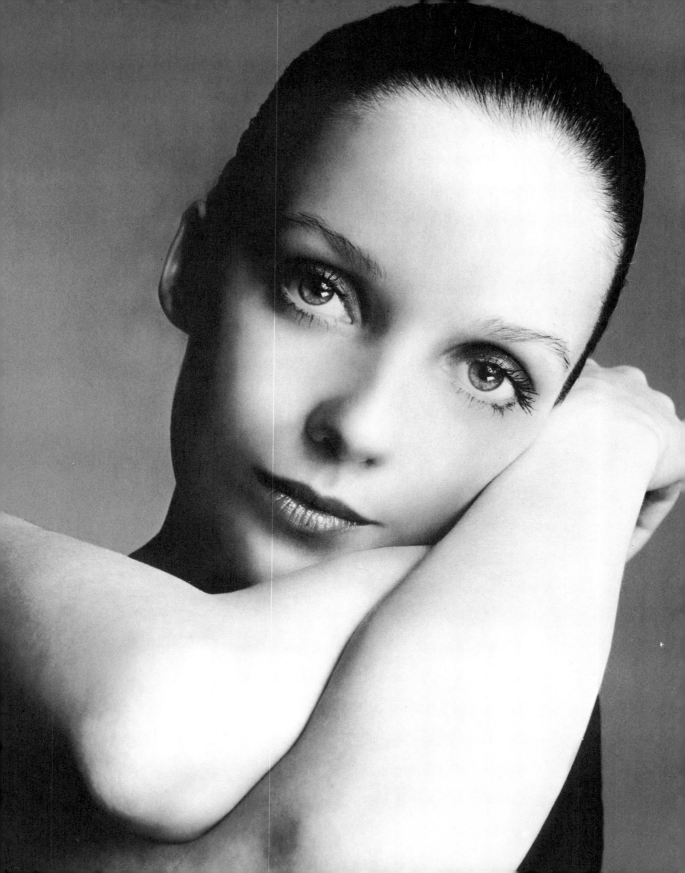

3

MIND AND MEDITATION

The subconscious and conscious mind together comprise the functional brain which operates twenty-four hours a day as a kind of computer, selecting and registering data and then feeding it back when we need it. Various philosophies hold that we also have a higher mind, a superconsciousness that has metaphysical powers and which, if harnessed, is capable of thought and action in a universal and spiritual way. Most of us are unaware of the existence of this cosmic mind, and do not understand it or know how to use it. During the past decade, however, the western world has shown increasing curiosity about it.

We have been greatly influenced by the teachings of the yoga philosophy, where complete detachment from reality, as we understand it, is the ultimate goal. The first step is to find 'self', because only by separating 'self' from the environment can one come to terms with individual personality and start putting the mind and emotions in order. This lack of self-knowledge is cited as the fundamental cause of many emotional and nervous problems; it is said to be responsible for the enormous discrepancy between our dreams and realities, which leads to frustration, tension, discontent, worry and finally physical illnesses.

The first move towards awareness of body and mind is achieved through the physical disciplines outlined in the previous chapter and through learning to relax. The next step is to become aware of controlling the mind through mechanical concentration. The third level is mastery of the mind through meditation, where insight can be gained into the cosmic mind, the ultimate 'self'. As you practise relaxation and concentration exercises, you learn to direct your thoughts and you become more aware of who and what you are. Without becoming either detached or indifferent, you will learn to be apart from your environment; people and things around you will cease to dominate your mind. You achieve a sense of freedom; you find strength within yourself to be yourself. All this releases tension and frees neuroses.

RELAXATION

Most of us are too tense; the human body was not made to cope with the stresses and strains of this age. There are a number of illnesses now considered to be psychogenic or psychosomatic – that is, originating in the psyche or mind – mostly triggered by our reaction to stress. For example, ulcers and colitis are nervous disturbances rare a generation ago; heart disease is more prevalent even in the relatively young; minor ills such as headaches, nervous fatigue, nervous indigestion, irritability, sleeplessness are only too common; and nothing consumes energy more than giving vent to emotions.

It is not easy to relax, yet it is clearly the first step to serenity and better health. The aim of relaxation is to quieten the nerves and relieve the body of all conscious tension and contraction. Relaxation can be learned; through it you can begin to handle both physical and mental problems more easily. Once you have discovered how to shut out the world around you for even a few minutes, you have a means of combating nervous fatigue and exhaustion.

There can be no physical relaxation without mental relaxation – and vice versa. To learn to relax completely takes practice and cannot be mastered in one easy lesson. You are not likely to achieve it on your first or even your second attempt. Deep relaxation is a conscious, willed process controlled by the mind, which in turn relaxes the body into complete immobility. It is widely assumed that to sleep is better than to relax. This is not so because, whereas during relaxation the mind is willing utmost repose, when asleep most of us continue to tense muscles unconsciously, often tossing and turning in agitation, which at times is caused by dreams. When starting a relaxation routine, habit is important. Try to do relaxing exercises at the same time every day – early morning, after work, late evening, for example. Clothes should be unrestricting, the fewer the better. This is the method:

Lie flat on your back on a carpet, rug or blanket on the floor, arms at sides. Take a few deep breaths.

Try to visualize the patterns of your muscles. Think of a coloured liquid being pumped along the muscle network. Now send mental messages along one of these 'roads', making muscles contract slowly; study what happens and think about it. Move limbs one at a time; flex a toe and notice a reflex movement in the thigh; stretch a finger and feel the progressive action. Then stretch the limbs, holding a moment to register sensations; let go. Repeat the process throughout the body until you are familiar with all muscle groups – neck, shoulders, back, abdomen.

Now stretch again, this time very slowly, beginning with the legs and arms, then the torso and finally the neck. Mentally visualize the muscle build-up. Hold the stretched position for a few seconds.

In slow motion, let go. This process is the basic mechanism of relaxation. The most effective way is to start at the top and work down; relax the head, the face, the eyes, the jaws, the mouth, the tongue, the neck and so on down to the toes. End up like a rag doll. Relax through mental willpower.

Now that you are completely at ease try to banish unnecessary thoughts from your mind. Stay relaxed as long as you can – fifteen minutes or so. The more you master the art, the deeper the degree of relaxation. As you become more proficient, you will find that you will not need to stay in the relaxed position so long: a ten-minute session will be enough.

To terminate relaxation, slowly restore control of each muscle group, starting with the toes and working your way up the body, finally stretching the neck and head. Conclude with a long cat-like stretch.

CONCENTRATION

This is the key to control of the mind and emotions. Our minds tend to be overloaded with trivia; in order to use our mental powers to the full, we have to learn to get rid of unnecessary thoughts and data. The aim of concentration is to achieve discipline and to harness mental energy so that daily activities may be done with increased efficiency.

For the Hindus, the goals are more ambitious; beginning with the art of concentration they attempt to achieve the state of *samadhi*, or super-consciousness, where the cosmic mind enters into the universe, into the Absolute spirit of life. This is done with the guidance of a guru, because such intense concentration – which is difficult to achieve alone – if undertaken without a mentor could result in either excessive dreaminess or such spiritual stimulus as to unbalance the mind.

Controlled concentration can improve memory and help to show you how to function at top capacity on intellectual and emotional levels. As with other personal disciplinary routines, it is important to practise concentration regularly, setting aside a specific time each day. In the early morning, late afternoon or at night before retiring are good times. After you have learned mind control, you will discover that thinking can be projected into sleeping hours, and you can train yourself to lodge any problems in the innermost mind – which continues to function during sleep – and awake refreshed and even aware of how to solve them.

The beginning of self-knowledge starts with mastery of concentration. Thinking becomes less muddled, you are less influenced by outside distractions and you begin to assess yourself honestly; tensions subside because you have cleared the mind of irrelevant trivia. There is no such thing as concentration in a mental vacuum; you must always concentrate on something. This is lesson number one, and must be mastered before further steps are taken. Focus your attention on something, an object or a mental image, shutting out everything else. The mind tends to wander, and undivided attention is difficult at first.

The following are simple exercises to teach you the art of concentration. They should be done quietly and alone; in comfortable clothes and position. Just as you had to learn to concentrate in order to relax, you now have to learn to relax in order to concentrate. You will be amazed how quickly you can train your mind to concentrate effectively, so that it will no longer wander when you have to focus on something specific in everyday affairs.

First an elementary concentration task. Sitting on the floor – cross-legged or in the Lotus position (see Movement, page 31) – look steadily at any object directly in your line of vision; absorb its form for about a minute. Now close the eyes and try to visualize the object in the space between your eyebrows. It will appear quite clear at first, then will begin to fade. Open your eyes and refresh your memory. Close your eyes and recall it.

Do this several times until you are able to hold the object visually in the mind for two minutes.

When walking down a street or entering a room, make yourself aware of surroundings; take everything in from a visual point of view; think of impressions. Afterwards, try systematically to recall as many visions as possible; push your memory.

The next step is to recall events. Start with thinking of yesterday. What did you do, what did you see? Don't just remember the highlights, make the mind re-enact events in their chronological order. It is interesting to notice what is overlooked at first; further mental probing will bring into focus incidental events. The mind records everything and concentration will bring complete recall.

Once the previous day's events are brought into general perspective, the next step is to recall and review the current day's happenings, constructively analysing behaviour and reactions before going to sleep. There are two difficulties here. First, because of tiredness the mind will want to wander; second, analysis of events of such proximity requires an honesty that is hard to achieve. However it is this very immediate confrontation that demands the utmost concentration and forces a self-examination that, if met with realism, is the giant step to self-knowledge.

MEDITATION

The preparatory disciplines of relaxation and concentration pave the way to true meditation. Once you are able to stay with a thought long enough to examine it closely before allowing the mind to go on to another subject, you have the self-control necessary for the final step. In meditation, instead of staying with one thought, the mind has to become a void through which thoughts are free to flow, calming the nerves, shutting out worry and eliminating negative attitudes. As you slowly master the art of meditation – and it is a slow process requiring perseverance – you will find that you are receptive to positive thoughts and ideas, and in so doing you re-educate the mind to work for you. In time you should be able to concentrate on whatever you want and discard unnecessary invasions swiftly. The positive outcome is that unfounded fears and worries can be pushed aside, failures are not dwelt upon, guilt feelings can be squashed and tension is reduced to a minimum.

The early days of meditation are trying. You feel self-conscious and inadequate as a thinker, but if you continue to practise only a few minutes a day, it can become a stimulating habit. Here are the guidelines:

It is essential to be alone and undisturbed. Shut yourself away in a quiet corner where there is no likelihood of interruption. Pick a time of day when there is little possibility of the phone ringing or the doorbell going.

It is traditional to sit in the classic Lotus Position, though cross-legged, tailor-fashion, is perfectly all right. Some people prefer to lie on their backs, arms alongside the body. It is essential to lie on a hard surface.

Correct rhythmic breathing is important (see Breathing, page 32) because it not only helps to put the body at ease but also brings the necessary *prana*.

Meditation may be begun by closing the eyes and trying to concentrate on a single part of the body. A common choice is that of the space directly above the bridge of the nose between the eyebrows; this is where the mystical 'third eye' is supposed to be. Think about it; imagine what it looks like and what it can see that the normal human eye cannot. Allow ideas and visions to come into the mind, all related to that third eye. Twelve seconds of such meditation is called *dharana*; if you manage to remain on that subject inviting more ideas for twelve times twelve seconds (almost two and a half minutes) you have achieved true meditation or *dhyana*.

Alternatively, meditate on the heart; think about what it looks like, its position, its beat, its function; feel your pulse to get its rhythm; now move away from the purely physical and dwell on the so-called emotions of the heart and develop thoughts as to why we associate the heart with love, happiness or distress.

Instead of looking inward, you can meditate on an external object; a candle or a light is often used. Concentrate on the candle for a minute, examining closely the form and colour of the light, the reflection of the wax. Palm your eyes and try to recall the candle; after a minute open the eyes and look more closely into it. Develop thoughts to do with light, the facts, the fantasies, the symbolic association of light with spirit. Any object can be meditated on in this way; elements of nature are good subjects – flowers, trees, clouds, a lake, the sea. You can also think of a person or a book.

Meditation can be practised through the sense of hearing; concentrate on a sound and direct all attention to it; it could be wind, rain, the lapping of water, the song of a bird, a waterfall, church bells. Again it is the flow of related thoughts that is the key to true meditation. A practical exercise is to listen to music for five minutes, imagining yourself as an instrument through which the music streams; concentrate on the sounds, the form of the music; just think of that particular music.

It is sometimes useful to meditate with the help of the voice, by repeating a *mantra* or sound. The most powerful one is said to be that of O . . . M. Inhale deeply, form the lips into an O and, keeping your voice low and steady, say the letter O until you have expelled half the air from the lungs; now close the lips and say the letter M, exhaling through the nose. Be aware of the sound vibrations. When all the air is used up, take a complete breath without pausing and repeat the exercise. Do this seven times.

All the senses can be used as agents for meditation, providing an almost endless range of subjects for single-minded thought. When you can achieve two or three minutes of such meditation, you can progress to a more advanced form, where the mind is shut off completely and no thoughts are allowed at all. Empty your mind of all distractions, all thoughts, and become conscious of what happens if you stop thinking altogether. When you are disturbed by a thought, push it firmly away; if you can achieve this for two or three minutes you will become aware of the usual turmoil the mind is in and the peace that comes from allowing it to rest.

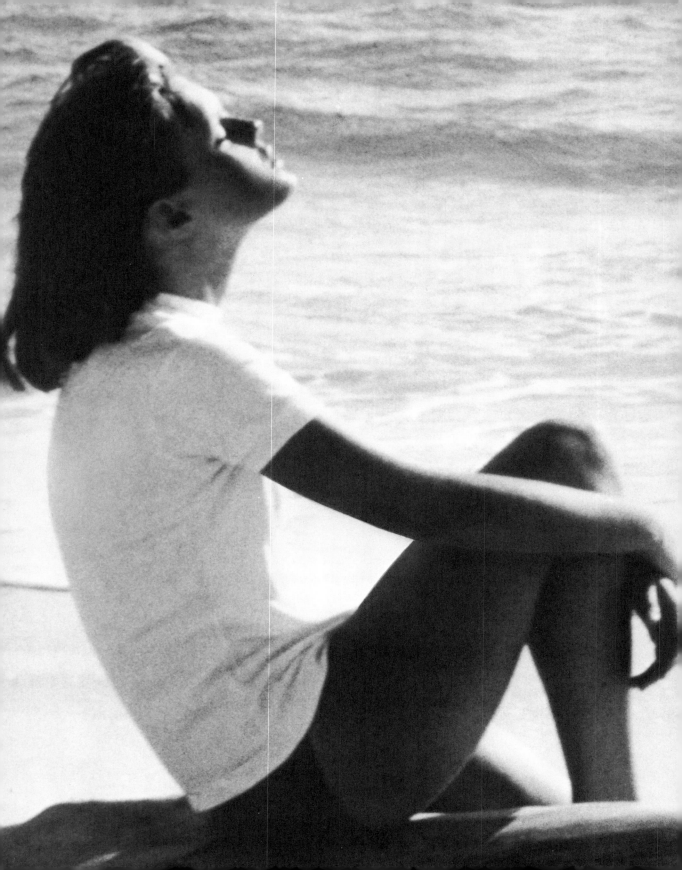

4

ENVIRONMENT

The atmosphere directly affects our health and attitudes, both beneficially and adversely. There is little, apart from heredity, that has so much influence on our general condition as the environment. Moods can be influenced by climate and latitude – warm, humid winds can depress, while long periods without rain make many people nervous. Be aware of the bad effects, and learn from the nature therapists how to benefit from the natural surroundings.

AIR

The air now contains an enormous number of polluting substances such as carbon monoxide, sulphur dioxide, fluorine, lead, dust particles and many chemicals and gases, and these are most hazardous in damp foggy environments. The increased ozone level of our immediate atmosphere is particularly hazardous as this gas often combines with other chemicals to form destructive compounds. Higher up, between fifteen and twenty miles above the earth, there is an ozone layer which protects us from most of the ultraviolet radiation from the sun; now this layer appears to be diminishing and there could be a danger of exposure to carcinogenic rays.

Air can pollute water, sea and land – and finally food. Pollution is the subject of much current research; not only is it getting worse, but researchers are constantly producing evidence that it is a contributory cause of many diseases, especially those of the respiratory tract and the circulation. Lungs provide the body with oxygen and eliminate the waste product, carbon dioxide; they also act as filters. Any damage to the lungs can therefore have far-reaching effects. We do not yet know the extent to which diseases are caused by air pollution; nor do we know how to combat it. Some experts say that certain vitamins and minerals may help, citing vitamin E in particular (a supplement of 100 i.u. a day) and suggest extra vitamin A, vitamin B–2 and B–3.

AIR TREATMENT

Pure air, however, is one of the important elements in all natural therapies. Clear, crisp mountain air or bracing sea air is the best. Air is important not just as the source of oxygen, but as a stimulus to the skin and, particularly, the activity of the sweat glands. Clothes should be porous to allow perspiration and preferably of natural fibre, wool, cotton and linen. Too much wrapping in wool, however, can cause the body to overheat, followed by the subsequent chilling evaporation of sweat. Synthetics trap air and hinder the skin's natural metabolism.

The humidity of the air is a significant factor. Dry, cold air is stimulating, for it speeds up body activity and circulation. Warm, moist air hinders perspiration (although intense moist heat, as in a Turkish steam bath, promotes it) and this prevents toxins from being released through the skin.

In natural therapy use is made of change from cold to warm and from dry to moist, both of which act as a stimulus. This is the principle behind the sauna treatment: a session in hot dry air, followed by a plunge in cold water or a roll in the snow (see page 64).

Air baths are recommended as a preventive measure to build up the body's natural resistance, as well as being indicated for specific ailments. They are said to be helpful in feverish conditions, in bronchitis (where the temperature of the air has to be professionally controlled), in kidney diseases and in some forms of arthritis. For healthy people, air baths can be taken out of doors, combined with exercise – such as walking or jogging in place. We should all expose our bodies to air more often: walking nude around the house, sleeping between cotton sheets without air-restricting synthetic nightwear, breathing deeply by an open window.

Exposure to cool air should be gradual, as not everyone has the ability to adapt immediately to the cold – the body should be partially exposed at first, and entirely bared later on. Air baths can be given in bed, as in many therapeutic centres, building up resistance. Air treatment is frequently combined with exposure to the sun – indeed is an integral part of it.

Temperature and altitude influence the composition of air and consequently its affect on the body. The rarified air of a higher altitude can be energizing up to the point where the oxygen content of the air is less and breathing becomes laboured.

We are adaptable to environment changes. It is true that some people function better in cold weather and others in hot, and this does not always depend on the climate in which you were brought up. The average body is capable of experiencing extremes of heat, cold and humidity without damage to health. Going from a very hot to a very cold climate has fewer problems than vice versa. Sleep is often affected – either you cannot sleep or you are constantly drowsy. Stomach upsets are common, which could be due to either nerves or a change of diet. But all these things are transitory and quickly adjusted.

SUN

It is a paradox that the sun is the best tonic for the whole body but in excess it can be a danger. Sunlight consists of several kinds of radiant energy: the visible rays that provide light, the infra-red rays that bring warmth and the ultraviolet rays that burn. Our first reaction to light is chemical and this then initiates a nervous response. The interaction between sun and skin is complex and it is therefore impossible to get tanned without getting burned unless adequate precaution is taken.

Sunlight enables the body to build up 75 per cent of its necessary store of vitamin D. Sunbathing for limited periods is also beneficial because the rays assist in the assimilation of calcium. It is thought, too, that sunlight might increase the efficiency of ovulation, thus accounting for the rise in the incidence of conception during summer months. Because the sun stimu-lates cell growth, resulting in a faster shedding of the old surface cells, unclogging pores and making them less vulnerable to infection, exposure to sunlight helps to clear up skin troubles.

A certain amount of sunlight – not necessarily concentrated exposure to the sun – is necessary for health. If too much time is spent in artificial light or in the dark, the production of cortisol, one of the essential hormones, is hindered. This affects the efficiency of night workers as it takes a minimum of ten days for the body to adjust to manufacturing cortisol during the hours of dark. The sun's energy is greatest early in the morning, *before* its rays reach their strongest, and natural therapists believe very much in this morning power for mental and physical build-up. Over-exposure to the sun's rays can atrophy and age the skin, finally resulting in cancer. It can also sterilize the skin to the point where many antibiotic micro organisms are destroyed and resilience to infection is therefore reduced. Some drugs – tranquillizers, contraceptives, antibiotics and antihistamines – make the skin unduly sensitive to the sun.

SUN TREATMENT

Sun treatment was very important before the discovery of antibiotic drugs, and is still widely used by natural practitioners. Dr A. Rollier in Switzerland pioneered sun treatment for tubercular patients; he not only cured their tuberculosis but improved their general health. There is no further need for this particular cure, but the principles of the Rollier approach remain the same. Rollier stressed the effect on the nervous system, starting in the nerve-endings of the skin and, through reflex action, stimulating the entire body and metabolism. Apart from its physiological effects, the sun relaxes and cheers the mind.

A sun treatment has to be taken gradually, three times a day. On the first day, expose the feet only for five minutes; on the second day bare the legs for five minutes, the feet for ten; on the third day, uncover the thighs for five minutes, the legs for ten minutes and the feet for fifteen. The strip-tease is continued until the entire body has been gradually exposed. Many people can stand the sun on the whole body from the start, provided the head is shaded, the sun not too hot and exposure begins at five or ten minutes and is gradually increased. This is the therapeutic way to get the sun – it is not the way to get a tan, though that will gradually build up. In high altitudes the sun's force is greater; reflections from sea, sand and snow intensify radiation, and exposure should be shorter. It is not necessary to lie down, provided the skin is directly exposed to the sunlight. This treatment can be done in low altitudes, but there the humidity and the higher proportion of cloudy days are a disadvantage. The Rollier technique can also be followed with an ultraviolet lamp, but only under professional supervision, as the time schedules have to be drastically modified.

WATER

Water cures have been practised for many years and their value is recognized in many quarters of the medical profession. Hydrotherapy has many facets: water as a beverage, baths, steam treatments, hot and cold compresses, underwater massage and internal irrigation all have their place in clinical régimes.

Therapeutic centres are usually concentrated in areas where special mineral waters are to be found. Many mineral waters are absorbed through the skin and have particularly beneficial effects on connective tissue. However, any water can be health-giving, providing it is fresh, clear and uncontaminated. Running water exposed to the sun is said to have special curative power (i.e., fast-flowing streams, moving lakes, open springs and pools where the water can absorb solar energy and pass it on to the body). This is not a new idea; the Greeks and Romans considered that the best self-cure was to drink from healing fountains where the gushing water had maximum exposure to air and sunlight.

Natural mineral waters are untreated, with nothing added and nothing removed. They can be still or sparkling – the latter found bubbling naturally from springs. No water is pure H_2O, but some natural waters have a combination of minerals that is palatable and good for the body. Hardness is determined by the acid–alkali balance; technically, pH7 indicates perfect neutrality, hard (alkaline) water has a pH value of over 7 and soft water a pH value of less than 7. Most bottled waters tend to be slightly alkaline (hard). Municipal waters can be hard or soft and are chemically purified by chlorination; fluorine may also be added, but this is considered to be a possible health hazard.

The importance of drinking a lot of water daily cannot be overstressed. Most spa cures emphasize it and, contradictory as it may appear, drinking a lot of water can reduce fluid retention – a freqent cause of overweight. This is because water is often held in the body by minerals and toxins, which need more water to swill them out. One of the advantages of learning to appreciate good water is to discover that it can be as satisfying as tea or coffee and for many it can serve instead of an aperitif. It is a taste worth acquiring.

Drinking is one thing, bathing another. 'Taking the waters' has been going on for hundreds of years, for it was known that sulphur water was good for sinews, alum waters helped paralysis, mud baths stimulated the nervous system, and so on. But it was not until the end of the nineteenth century that water treatments as we know them today were initiated, when the therapeutic benefits of ordinary water were realized. Priessnitz of Austria pioneered the way by using cold applications to help stimulate the vital organs and detoxify the body; he employed showers, total immersion, partial baths, packs with wet sheets and compresses – all very cold. Father

Kneipp is probably one of the best-known water doctors; he believed that fresh cool living water contained great healing power and preached the benefits of living a simple life in the fresh air.

COLD-WATER TREATMENT

The body responds to a cold stimulus by producing its own heat, which automatically increases the blood supply. Many therapists swear by the value of cold treatment and use nothing else. The various skin and body types differ in their reaction to the cold. Chubby people tolerate it well, the slender need gradual build-up, the athletic can stand only infrequent, though forceful, applications. If the skin glows on sudden exposure to cold water, the body will respond well to treatments; if it blanches, it will not. There are several types of cold-water therapy. Since the end of the last century naturopaths have advocated these treatments, which do not get the backing of today's medical practitioners, but which are said to invigorate, stimulate and bring relief to certain conditions.

Exercise

This is a method of hardening the system, not treating maladies. The idea was originated by Father Kneipp. It consists of walking barefoot in wet grass for 15–45 minutes a day (it makes no difference if the grass is wet from dew, rain or watering), in freshly fallen snow for 3–15 minutes, on wet stones for 3–5 minutes or in cold water first to the ankle, then to the knee, for 1–6 minutes. Immediately afterwards, dry socks and shoes must be put on without drying the feet; then a brisk walk of 10 minutes, fast at first and slowing down to normal speed.

Compress

The cold-water compress causes perspiration and helps to eliminate toxic matter. A piece of linen is wrung out in cold water and applied to specific areas, covered with layers of wool or blankets so as to exclude air. The degree of stimulus is decided by the thickness of the wet layer and the position of the compress. It is essential to be warm before and after the application of the compress so as to encourage perspiration. A warm bath is sometimes taken before treatment. The compress is left in position until sweating stops. The wet layers are removed, but the patient remains wrapped in a blanket. At this point a milder form of sweating may result;

when that is finished the blanket is lifted away, and the body sponged with cold water and dried. An upper compress stretches from the neck to the base of the spine or abdomen. A lower compress usually goes from the armpits to the hips and can strengthen the spine, bringing relief to back pains. There are compresses for specific areas – neck, hands, arms, feet, leg and the pelvic region. A stomach compress is good for pains, cramp and congestion of the heart and chest; a cold compress on the head will relieve a headache due to fever.

Packing

This consists of enveloping whole areas in a wet sheet, covered with a blanket. The swathing is kept in position from thirty minutes to a couple of hours depending on the condition. If you are healthy it can be kept on all night. It benefits liver and kidneys and brings relief to heart and stomach troubles and flatulence. An alternative is to wear a wet shirt with the same blanket covering; the shirt may be kept on for one to two hours; this is particularly good for soothing the nervous system and is valuable in many skin diseases as it draws poisons to the surface. The shirt can be dipped in a mixture of vinegar and water.

Affusion

This is a bracing and invigorating shower of cold water sprayed on specific areas from a watering can or hose: from knee to feet, from neck to waist, from the nape of the neck to the coccyx, the whole body. A healthy person will benefit from cold showering, but invalids should use tepid water.

Bathing

The stimulus of the cold bath varies according to the area of the skin immersed. The cold footbath consists of putting the feet and legs up to or above the calves in cold water, for one to three minutes. This draws blood away from the head and chest; it is invigorating for the limbs and can relieve fatigue. In the cold sitz bath – lasting from $\frac{1}{2}$ to 3 minutes – the water covers the upper part of the thigh to the middle of the abdomen; the legs should be left free and dry. It is a particularly valuable water application; it helps to regulate circulation, cures constipation, expels gases and alleviates hae-morrhoids. It can also stimulate the reproductive organs and the spine. The body must be warm before taking the plunge and you may perspire during the bath. Afterwards dress quickly without drying and exercise until the body has regained its normal temperature. Take no more than three cold baths a week.

HOT-WATER TREATMENT

This promotes sweating and may be applied to the whole body or parts of it as moist or dry heat. Neither the steam bath nor the sauna should be taken until an hour after eating, nor while under the influence of alcohol or drugs.

Steam Bath

The temperature can be raised to a high level as long as the head is kept cool. There are special cabinets that enable the body to be exposed to steam at a temperature of 120°F (49°C), while the air inhaled is kept down to 26°F ($-$3°C). In this way the body can reach a level of maximum perspiration, while the blood vessels in the brain remain normal. Beneficial effects are said to be: removal of toxic substances, reduction of blood sugar, lowering of cholesterol, decrease of carbon monoxide and increase of oxygen in superficial venous blood, removal of ammonia from the tissues and greater fluidity of blood.

The Sauna

The whole body is exposed to dry heat with occasional blasts of moist air for ten minutes. The temperature is higher than that of the moist bath – anywhere from 100–200°F (38–93°C). The dry heat is followed by exposure to cool air or cold water for fifteen minutes, then a rest for an additional fifteen minutes. The change from heat to cold is the significant factor, as it can help regulate blood pressure, thereby helping circulation and the heart. Perspiration aids the elimination of toxic matter, and the whole process is particularly invigorating and stimulating. It is essentially for healthy people; older people, and those suffering from diabetes, heart disease and high blood pressure, should not take sauna baths; for everyone, the timing must be controlled.

Local Applications and Baths

Lint hot-water compresses are used to treat contaminated cuts and wounds or to draw out poisonous or foreign matter. A hot arm bath is helpful in angina pectoris as it relaxes the arteries and improves the blood supply to the heart. Warm footbaths are for people in a weak condition and with poor circulation; they make the blood flow to the feet and have a sedative action; they are helpful in headache, sore throat and cramp conditions.

COLD AND HOT COMBINATIONS

This involves some areas of the body being exposed to cold, others to hot; this type of therapy is generally controlled by a qualified practitioner as a number of problems are invariably involved. However, exposing the body to alternate hot and cold waters is something everyone can practise to stimulate health and vigour. The combination sitz bath is popular for toning up the pelvic region. Two tubs are needed, one with the temperature at 50–65°F (10–18°C), the other pleasantly hot. First sit in the hot water for ten to fifteen minutes, then in the cold for only half a minute; make three or four changes in this way, always finishing with the cold bath. Any small tub can be used, but if you prefer the bath, fill it with water about 10 in. (25 cm.) high and sit in it with the knees drawn up; if there is no large tub for the cold water, wash the body quickly under a cold shower or use a sponge and cold water. Take ten minutes for the hot relaxing soak and one minute only for the bracing cold, three times each, ending with the cold. In fact, it is healthier to end any bath with a quick cold sponging.

SEA

Salty sea water is extremely rich in minerals and over sixty elements have been discovered in it. The minerals are thought to act as catalysts to improve body metabolism.

Sea air is high in fortified oxygen molecules that act as a disinfectant for the whole body – deep breathing can revive the whole circulatory system.

The use of sea water internally is not so well known. In ionized form it is readily assimilated by the body. Some naturopaths recommend drinking 1 oz. (30 g.) daily to obtain the trace amounts of minerals the body requires.

Large areas of sea water are now polluted, but uncontaminated sea water can be obtained from health stores. It has proved effective for digestive troubles and weakened constitutions; compresses will help burns, sores and boils. Haemorrhoids and other rectal problems have been aided with sea water enemas.

EARTH (CLAY)

The healing properties of clay have been known for centuries. Some areas produce particularly potent mud (see pages 91–2) often of volcanic origin, powerful enough to get limbs moving after accidents and subsequent atrophy. Clay is extremely absorbent, drawing out impurities from the body; it is also antiseptic and naturally preserves important body flora while combating infection. It contains a very high percentage of silica, which makes it suitable for treating ageing and a large variety of degenerative disorders. It has appreciable amounts of magnesium, iron and lime–calcium, which means it is useful for mineral deficiency and anaemia.

Clay is now used externally and internally. For external application it is made into a paste by adding water; the consistency should be quite thick so that it will adhere to the skin. It can be applied directly to the skin – cold, tepid or warm: cold for the treatment of inflammation of the lower abdomen; lukewarm or hot for liver, kidney, bladder or bones. When used for varicose veins it is sometimes applied as a compress.

Many clinics and health farms have mud baths and treatments. Applications may be left from one to three hours and sometimes overnight. Abscesses and infections need hourly changes in the early stages. Initial applications are thinner than the final ones.

It is possible to make a mud bath at home: The clay is mixed with warm water until it is muddy but not slimy. The initial immersion should be for five or ten minutes only, followed by baths of fifteen to twenty every second or third day for a month. Do not repeat the series until another month has elapsed. A mud bath is good for arthritis and rheumatism; partial baths can be used to relieve the hands or feet.

Clay is also employed for vaginal douches and enemas, helping colitis, intestinal disorders and vaginal infections. Use three to four tablespoons to a quart (1 l.) of water.

Internally, clay stimulates lethargic body organs and metabolism, yet the chemical analysis alone does not explain the extent of its curative properties. It is capable of re-establishing a stable equilibrium by giving a push to deficient glandular function and it also fights germs.

Green, white, yellow or red clay can be used after being freed of any sand or impurities. One teaspoon of clay is mixed in a teacup of water; it is normally taken on rising, but also can be drunk half an hour before a main meal or at bedtime. A stronger dose of two to three teaspoons is needed for anaemia, dysentery and colitis. Take daily doses for three weeks, and for ten days a month thereafter.

SPACE

The way your body reacts to time and space is an individual relationship with the environment and the universe. Although the body can adjust quite rapidly to climate change, it is not so adept at adapting to upsets in the twenty-four-hour time-cycle. Swift travel from one time-zone to another unbalances the whole biological clockwork and affects metabolism as well as mental responses.

Journeys following the lines of longitude do not provide so many problems even though climatic change may be drastic. Stress, due only to displacement and the physical aspects of travel, is limited. You can expect fatigue and some tension, but the body rhythm will tick along as usual.

Travelling along the lines of latitude is different. Studies reveal that adjustment to a new time-zone takes at least five days going east to west and seven days going west to east. The circadian rhythm is very disturbed; depression, moodiness, tension and strain invariably result; soundness of judgement is lowered and physical ability is under par. The zone-change syndrome is real, and is not merely due to travel fatigue. The body has to get into its new gear of sleeping, waking and eating.

Physically and psychologically we are very much tied to the sequences of the sun and moon – and other planets. Menstrual cycles, for example, are lunar; daily metabolism is affected by the solar day. Most people have more active heart rates at noon and higher hormone production at sunrise; during the night the body repair work increases – cells are renewed, proteins remade, the nervous system recharged. Drugs often react differently according to the time of day. Different people may have different timing, but it is regular. Our relationship with the environment goes very deep; we can use it to our benefit if we seek the pure and remain aware of increasing daily contamination.

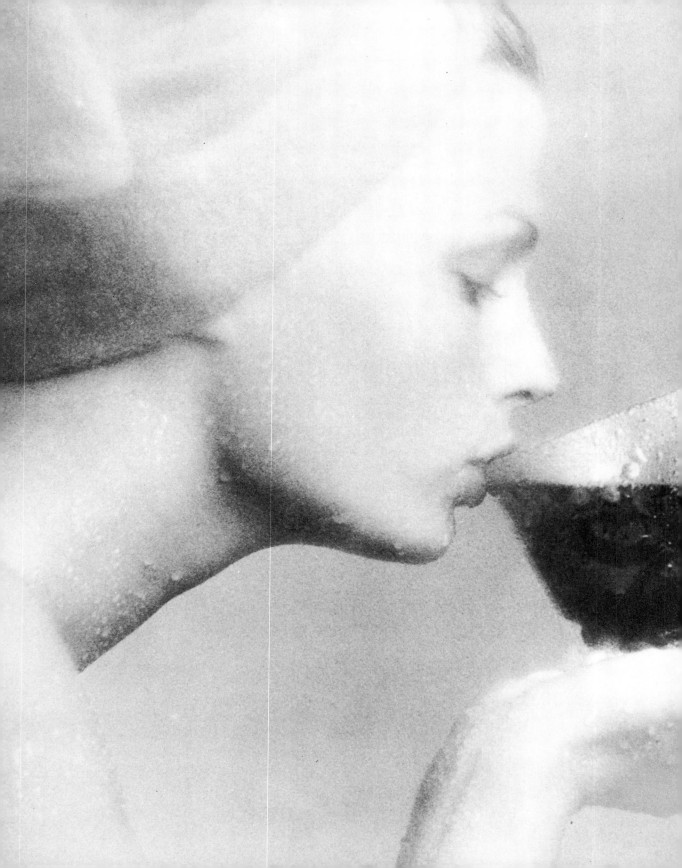

5

NATURAL THERAPEUTICS

What we call orthodox medicine is allopathy, which works by a process of analysis and deals with problems by isolating them. Any disorder is generally treated by chemical intervention or surgery. Allopathy has gained prominence over the last hundred years as we have learnt how to use drugs more effectively and surgery has become safer. The principles of the alternative medical therapies are diverse, but in general the whole person – body, mind and spirit – is treated. Much alternative medicine is preventive and self-corrective; it uses the many aspects of nature and the environment to achieve its end.

There are a surprising number of natural therapies, many complementary to each other and often used in conjunction. Some systems date back thousands of years – acupuncture, for instance – while others, particularly in the energy field, are relatively recent. They may be divided into three main groups: organic, spiritual and the use of cosmic energy. All are auxiliaries to conventional medicine, not substitutes for it. Practitioners of any of the following principles are realistic enough to accept that they are but part of the broad spectrum of medical aid. While it is correct to trust the healing power of nature, it cannot be considered infallible. Virulent infections and germs will respond only to antibiotics; surgery is sometimes unavoidable; metabolic failures may require artificial or chemical substitutes. It is, however, well worth investigating the curative possibilities provided by nature; ideally this should be the first move, not the last resort. The following is a summary of the most important alternative treatments, explaining the theories and the methods.

ACUPUNCTURE

A standard form of medical treatment in China for thousands of years, now being adopted as a therapy by many western physicians. The basic principle is that energy – the life force – flows through certain channels in the body; if this flow is interrupted or diminished, pain or illness occurs.

It is thought that acupuncture began when men became aware of the sensitivity of certain parts of the skin when the body was out of order in some way. In time, certain points were linked to specific illnesses. There are approximately 800 of these points over the body, forming a definite pattern; the lines that connect particular organs with these points are called meridians. These are energy pathways, the route of *ch'i*, the life force. Acupuncturists believe that health exists only when this energy flows freely and is in a state of perfect balance; excess or deficiency leads to a metabolic disorder. Balance depends on the two energies of *yang* and *yin* – the positive and negative forces, as in electricity.

The art of the acupuncturist lies in his ability to smooth the energy flow in the meridians. He tries to redistribute the energies by lightly inserting needles of pure copper, silver or gold at specific points along the meridian lines. The gold needles act as a stimulant, the silver ones sedate. Very slender needles are used, in numbers varying from two or three to a dozen or more. Often there is no feeling when needles are inserted, sometimes a slight tingling. The amount of time they are kept in place depends upon the disorder – for example, ten minutes to help relieve headaches.

Through experience it is possible to tell by touch which points need to be treated. A pulse diagnosis is fundamental in acupuncture; a practitioner is trained to feel fourteen pulses above the wrist, and is able to detect any excess or depletion of energy. So sensitive are these pulse readings, that not only can past illnesses be revealed, but it is possible to forecast disorders long before physical symptoms appear. This makes acupuncture particularly valuable as a preventive therapy. On a curative level, a series of treatments are usually necessary.

Conditions which can be successfully treated include migraine, head-ache, ulcers and digestive troubles, lumbago, arthritis, fibrositis, neuritis, sciatica, rheumatism, dermatitis, eczema and other skin conditions, asthma and bronchitis, anxiety and depression. In Chinese hospitals it is used not only as a therapy but it is also used instead of an anaesthetic during operations.

BIO-FEEDBACK

The easiest way to explain bio-feedback is to say that it is a method of training the mind to control body functions that are usually involuntary. Bio-feedback has recently revealed that we can control our physical condition to a degree that had previously seemed impossible, though no one really knows how it works. There are a number of mechanical techniques involved; the most basic is the monitoring of electrical skin resistance by using a device attached to the palms or fingertips of the hand. This measures the galvanic skin response, or amount of perspiration on the skin; it is not the apparent wetness or dryness of the hand that is tracked, but the changes of polarization at the sweat gland membranes, and this is determined by the blood flow rate. It is a way of establishing how tense or relaxed the body is, a vital link in the cause and cure of many disorders resulting from a block in the stress–relaxation mechanism.

Daily pressures of any kind trigger the fight-or-flight response, which is totally automatic: heart rate is increased, blood pressure goes up, blood goes to the muscles where tension is increased, the cortisone level in the blood rises and the digestive system shuts off. All this happens very quickly and the body's natural counteraction is the relaxation response, which eventually returns the body systems to normal. However, this balancing response is frequently incomplete, leaving a state of partial tension and this is where the trouble starts: continuing high blood pressure can overburden the heart, constantly tensed muscles cause fibrositis, a partially working digestive system encourages ulcers and unused cortisone reduces the body's immunity to disease.

It is clearly bad to stay in a state of partial tension for a long time and normal relaxation response can be learned through bio-feedback training. Under-responsive people can become more alert and active, over-responsive personalities can learn to be more calm and relaxed.

The monitoring device is usually attached to a machine which translates the electrical information into visible or audible forms – a light or a buzz. The brighter the light or the louder the buzz, the stronger the fight-or-flight reaction. Because instruction can become involved and unclear, the usual arrangement is simply to connect the bio-feedback device, with the instruction to stop the light or the buzz. As you have no idea how to do it, experiments begin. You can tense muscles but the noise or light becomes more forceful. You can relax and the buzz or light diminishes, but does not disappear. What next? Now the mind is put to test; you think of ways to almost will extinction; you think of people, things, scenes, events, colours ... Suddenly the light goes out or the buzzing stops. What caused that? If the same thought process is recalled and repeated – and with the same result – bio-feedback has worked. The device is then usually adjusted to a greater degree of sensitivity, thus bringing control to a finer degree.

Once you learn how to become deeply relaxed, the same state of mind can engineer the process without the use of a device or machine. Sometimes bio-feedback is used not to teach relaxation, but to gain control over muscles. Here, devices measuring slight muscular activity are attached to the part of the body in question. Instead of turning off the machine, it turns it on. This is very valuable in cases of paralysis and in the rehabilitation of stroke and accident victims.

Bio-feedback is being used in hospitals to supplement or eliminate other treatments. It is effective for migraine and headaches caused by tension, for high blood pressure, for gastric and duodenal ulcers, for retraining of muscles and for a wide range of nervous disorders resulting from modern stress. It is effective in the prevention of these disorders, because if the mind can be trained, the body will be healthier.

When bio-feedback is taught along with yoga or meditative relaxation (see pages 29ff. and 49ff.) the results are often quicker. It is a natural therapeutic measure as only body power is used; the monitoring machines merely act as vehicles of registration and mental stimulation.

BIO-RHYTHMS

These are the individual's variations in mood and performance relating to fluctuating supplies of energy. If you know your bio-rhythms you can take advantage of energy peaks – go with the tide rather than against it. We have three basic energy cycles: the physical cycle, which has a twenty-three day span and controls vitality, stamina and general health; the emotional cycle, which covers twenty-eight days and affects moods, creativity and emotional reactions; and the intellectual cycle, which has a rhythm of thirty-three days and controls mental ability, concentration and rationality.

Each cycle has an active phase when energy is flowing freely, a passive stage when there is less energy, and transition periods, where energy ebbs and flows and is generally unstable. All cycles commence at birth. There are periods, of course, when all three cycles are simultaneously at a zenith;

energy abounds, and unless it is all spent these periods can be the most disturbing of all and you can feel irritable, on edge, nervous, tense and at times depressed.

Bio-rhythms only reveal the pattern of variation in energy; your reaction to it depends upon your character, genes, environment and current situation. It is possible to obtain charts of bio-rhythms and calculate your own schedule, which will reflect your moods and behaviour. It can be used as a way of getting the most out of yourself mentally, physically and emotionally. You can take advantage of available energy and avoid overtaxing the system when it is at a low. You can push yourself during active phases and just maintain yourself during passive ones. If you learn the pattern of your bio-rhythms, the information can be related to daily living and personal relationships; it provides an opportunity to make the best of your abilities and it can also reduce tension and frustration.

CHIROPRACTIC

The relationship between bones and nerves is the underlying principle of chiropractic – the belief that disease is not only an entity that invades the body, but can be caused by neuro-irritations stemming from deranged muscles and joints. Attention is concentrated on the spine because this is the main connective centre for the nervous system. Pressure, strain or tension upon the spinal cord, caused by segments of the vertebral column being out of place, affect nerve transmission. Minor subluxations (misalignments) through an accident or merely through faulty posture can cause nerve inflammation and block the nerve passages. This results in an unhealthy state in the organs of the body controlled by the nerves in question.

The chiropractor manipulates the joints of the body, particularly the spinal vertebrae, to restore normal placement and function of the joints and the related nerve network, and thus restore health. The correction is carried out with repeated thrusts, rather than with a continuous kneading movement.

On consultation, a chiropractor will first ask for the history of the case in the normal way. A standard physical examination is given, plus a thorough and precise probing of the spinal column, pelvis, posture and muscle areas relating to the pain pattern. The use of radiography is especially important, and X-rays are studied to find out the extent of bone deviation or lesion. To help confirm findings, a chiropractor often uses a machine which monitors small differences in temperature along the spinal column: the inflammation set up by the lesions is said to produce a small degree of heat.

It is difficult to indicate how much treatment is necessary and how often. In many acute cases success is quick, depending on age. In chronic conditions with other complications, the response may be very slow or even totally absent.

What conditions can chiropractic help? Firstly, it is a notable preventive measure, since health depends very much on a good transmission of nervous energy. In general the following disease patterns respond well: spinal lesions associated with muscular pains, neuritis, neuralgia, sciatica, rheumatic and arthritic conditions, migraine, headaches, high and low blood pressure, some asthmas and certain nervous complaints due to stress. A chiropractor invariably employs auxiliary naturopathics – diet, posture correction, remedial exercise, massage, physiotherapy, water/heat/light therapies, acupressure and yoga for breathing and relaxation.

COLOUR THERAPY

The Egyptians and Persians used colour therapy extensively but, although it is known that colour affects us both physically and mentally, little use has been made of it in contemporary medical practice. Recently, renewed interest has been shown, particularly now that it is possible to measure the effects of light on living matter. For instance it has been scientifically established that blue light is calming, red light stimulating.

Colour is light of a specific wave length. The visible spectrum goes from red (the longest waves that the eye can see) to violet (the shortest); green is more or less in the middle and the human eye responds to it the least.

The effect of colour on the body is controlled by the nervous system which triggers both mental and physical responses. Although the reaction varies according to the individual the general effect is the same. Colour is also form, intensity and substance, and together they provide a medium for colour to become visible. It is this combination, at times used in rhythmic applications, that can instigate harmony or tension. The effect of the seven main colours and the many shades in between can be part of an overall health-maintenance pattern and is frequently taken into consideration in decorating and lighting clinics and medical centres.

Colour therapy can be both preventive and curative. Sensitive instruments have registered the lowering of blood pressure under blue light and the raising of blood pressure under red light. It can sometimes provide emergency aid; for example, during an asthmatic attack a blue light will lower tension, thus relaxing the muscles and bringing relief. At the moment there are only a few colour-therapy centres, where specialized treatment is given through a device called the Colour-Form-Rhythm Beamer. It is important to use the three complementary elements; colour comes through a lens-like window and is beamed in rhythmic timing, increasing and decreasing in strength according to individual needs. A treatment session lasts about twenty minutes; one to four treatments a week is usual.

COPPER PROTECTION

People suffering from rheumatism, lumbago, sciatica and arthritis have found relief from wearing an item of copper next to the skin – a bracelet, a watch-strap lining, a necklace. It seems extraordinary that such a simple device works, but thousands of copper wearers swear by it. It not only helps, but it takes effect very quickly. Whether it works on a preventive level is hard to determine, but many people wear a copper band 'just in case'.

Its current use originated in South Africa, where it was discovered that tribesmen who wore copper – at times a considerable amount – were free from aches and pains. The puzzle was – how did it work? Research revealed rheumatic sufferers had a copper deficiency, and it may be that this can be adjusted by osmosis through the skin from an external copper source.

EYE TRAINING

The theory that vision defects are irreversible because of the deterioration of the eye's lens was disproved more than fifty years ago. All credit is due to an American eye physician, Dr William H. Bates, who, by the time he died in 1931, had brought a whole new dimension to eye treatment and cure to many thousands. His system had remarkable results but was never taken up by the profession on the whole, although individuals who have diligently followed his methods are amazed at the improvement.

He asserted that the process controlling both near and distant vision was not – as is generally accepted – a function of the lens, but of two oblique extrinsic muscles encircling the eyeball. He argued that eye muscles like any other muscles can be trained. This is the basis of the Bates method. It can correct in part or totally the following problems: short-sightedness, defective sight due to old age, vision that is not clear (either near or far), astigmatism (where sight is blurred or distorted) and squinting.

The eye is retrained by first learning to relax, and then finding automatic responses naturally and gradually. There are a number of fundamental steps to be taken:

Palming: Relax by closing the eyes. Because light can penetrate the lids, it is important to cover the eyes with the palms of the hand, fingers crossing on the forehead and giving pressure there instead of on the eyeballs. Relax in this way for a few minutes when the eyes feel tired, or at intervals during the day.

Swinging: The eye usually remains fixed on a point for a fraction of a second only; if longer the eye is strained and vision impaired. To teach the eye to dart from one point to another, Dr Bates found body swinging useful, the reason being that the rhythm of the movement is gradually transmitted to the nerves controlling the extrinsic eye muscles. If done for a long enough time, the eye automatically takes up the pattern.

To swing, stand with feet a little apart, turning on the left foot to move the body to the right, then swing to the left side using the right foot as a pivot. The head and shoulders should be aligned, and only the body moved, not the eyes; be careful not to watch anything in particular. The stationary objects around you will appear to move. Swing for a minimum of five minutes at a time.

Blinking: The normal eye blinks gently and frequently; a faulty eye rarely. Force the eyes to blink, training them to make this gesture automatically. The exercise itself can often clear vision, if only for a moment.

Sunning: Sunlight is as necessary to a normal eye as relaxation. This does not mean looking into the sun – this is dangerous. Allow the sun to warm the closed lids for a minute or two, moving the face from side to side so that the sun is not concentrated on one spot. Afterwards, palm the hands over the eyes to shut out the light for a moment. It is interesting to note in this connection that people who live in sunny climates have fewer eye deficiencies, and it is now thought this may be due to the constant exercise necessary to adjust from bright sunlight to shadow.

Time is necessary to benefit from the Bates's eye-training technique, but diligent application can bring amazing results. Tense and nervous personalities require more time than those who have a calm temperament.

FAITH HEALING

The remarkable achievements of faith – or spiritual – healing can be explained in terms of cosmic energy. The healer acts as a vehicle for the accumulation and transfer of this energy to the patient. How it works is a mystery; lack of scientific explanation, however, cannot belittle the impressive results. We do not understand why gravity or magnetism work either, but accept that they do. Faith healing claims to have helped very nearly every type of condition, from headaches to heart attacks, arthritis, disabilities and inoperable conditions, including malignancies.

The charged particles of energy are known to the eastern yogis as *prana* and to the western world as the universal life force. This energy surrounds us, flowing freely in space, but it can be harnessed by certain people who use it for healing. A healer often sensitizes himself by certain occult practices: these can include deep breathing, the uttering of a mantra, meditation, sound vibrations and prayer. It is said that thought and concentration can summon and direct energy.

Healing power does not just appear – it comes from hard work on the healer's part. Discipline of daily life is stressed, as this leads to learning; breathing and meditation are the two significant ways of achieving the necessary control of the physical body, mind and thoughts.

The most prevalent method of healing involves the manipulation of energy through the hands into the psychic centres of the patient. It is explained that this passes through openings in the human aura (see page 81); in reverse the magnetism of the healer draws out the disease condition, pulling it free from the encircling aura. Hands are placed near or on the body; healing is done through the fingers or the palms. It is essential that the healer is completely relaxed and does not consciously direct energy to any single spot. The hands must be free to move where they want, and only experience can tell when they are in positive positions.

Sensations in the patient vary; many feel nothing, others are ultrasensitive, often feeling hot or cold in the areas being healed – and invariably the healer's hands feel the opposite. There can be tingling, prickling, pains and even a creaking of joints. The hands are kept in place until sensation ceases; sometimes when a condition is well advanced there is no sensation, in which case several healing sessions are necessary.

Faith healing has been successful when conducted from a distance and this is probably the most baffling of all phenomena in this field. There are even reports of health improving immediately after a letter has been written requesting help – before the healer has received it.

Conventional medicine cannot account for the successes. The formal attitude is to label them 'spontaneous remissions' which is a general excuse for any earlier diagnosis or doom pronouncements. However, practitioners of other forms of natural therapeutics are beginning to accept that a healing force, a bio-energy element, may be at work in their treatments. This is leading to mutual collaboration and the employment of a wide range of therapies conducted 'in faith'.

HERBALISM

Only medicines obtained from plants are used. This is the principle that separates herbalism from allopathy, though both aim to heal through admitting outside substances to the body. Allopathy uses chemicals or isolated botanical extracts, herbalism uses the whole plant wherein is packaged a complexity of natural elements – proteins, enzymes, minerals, chlorophyll, vitamins, terpenoids, polycelluloses, glucosides and phenols. The lack of toxicity in herbal remedies is believed to be due to the interaction of the active parts, where one element backs up the work of another. This is called synergism; joint effort of this kind is absent in synthetic reproductions. When analysed as separate entities, many of the component parts of a particular herb appear to be inert, yet herbalists maintain that their mere presence is significant, perhaps as a vital catalyst. Another argument is that these passive elements may be there as a buffer, as agents to help modify the harsh action of the active part.

Herbs not only cure diseases; their preventive role is also of tremendous importance. For details of self-help on both levels see Herbs and Tisanes, pages 117ff.

On a professional basis, symptoms are treated with specific herbs, but diagnosis involves the entire physical person and personality. Methods of consultation and diagnosis vary between practitioners. Usually the conventional stethoscope and a blood-pressure gauge are used. Certain analytical tests are taken, the most common being that of the urine. Confidence between the practitioner and patient is a significant factor, and it is important that a patient continues with the same practitioner; lasting benefit can only come from continuity. Disorders respond in different ways: some respond quickly, others require many months and an illness may very well get worse before getting better – but that is often the course of natural therapeutics.

Herbal remedies are neither toxic nor habit-forming. They are given in the form of pills, capsules, juices, extracts or ointments; they may be made from one or several herbs, ground to powder, potentized in liquid, or made into infusions, which can be done at home.

Herbalism provides remedies for almost every disorder of the body. In some cases it can replace surgery: those involving ulcers, gallstones, malignancies and advanced infections. Disorders of the entire digestive and respiratory system respond very well to herbal treatment, also nervous complaints, urinary difficulties, skin diseases, arthritis and rheumatism. In all instances, no matter what degree of improvement is attained, at least there is no risk of the harmful side-effects often associated with chemical drugs.

HOMOEOPATHY

To become an homoeopathic practitioner, it is necessary to first qualify as a physician. There are four major differences between conventional medicine and the homoeopathic approach to illness. Firstly, homoeopathy treats the whole person, not isolated symptoms, and a remedy is selected to match the total condition. Secondly, the drug chosen is based on its ability to provoke a similar set of reactions if given to a healthy person: this is the principle of like cures like. Thirdly, remedies are from natural not chemical sources – they are derived from the vegetable, animal and mineral worlds – and have no side-effects. Fourthly, remedies are given in highly diluted form, as it has been found that the curative action is increased this way.

Homoeopathy was originated by a German physician, Samuel Hahnemann, at the end of the nineteenth century. He was exceedingly thorough in his initial 'provings' of drugs, trying them on himself and others. Recently many of his early remedies have been 're-proved' and in all cases the efficacy of the original work has been endorsed. Today there are about 2,000 medicines in the homoeopathic materia medica.

It is a comprehensive and flexible list, and is used by many practitioners in other branches of alternative medicine, particularly on a preventive level. There are also about twenty remedies, covering most of the common ailments, which are available from a few specialized pharmacies for first aid and self-medication.

Homoeopathy is essentially an individual treatment; maladies can only be cured after careful history-taking and observation of symptoms. Reaction to environment and circumstances is considered to be as significant as organic manifestations. All patients show a slightly different symptom picture even if the illness is basically the same. Take a cold, for instance; this may come out as a fever, sore throat, runny eyes, nose blockage or discharge; one patient may feel better in fresh air, another in a hot bath, another in a warm room. One may feel thoroughly miserable and irritable, another only slightly put out. All aspects are taken into consideration. No single remedy could possibly appease all symptom variations and therefore the remedy or remedies that produce 'similar' results are selected according to the individual case. The other diagnostic methods follow the conventional routine of physical examination, pulse rate, temperature, blood pressure, urine and blood analysis.

Because of the nature of homoeopathic remedies, they can be of particular value in nervous conditions, where the origin of illness is undefinable.

Although science cannot fully explain why homoeopathic treatment works, there is a parallel between it and the orthodox application of vaccination, inoculation and immunization. Here a very small, modified quantity of the disease is used to prevent or combat its possible invasion of the body by stimulating natural defences. It would seem logical that homoeopathy works in much the same way – mobilizing the body's natural fighting agents.

This way of healing may be much slower than the allopathic one. A chronic condition takes longer than an acute illness, simply because it is more deeply rooted. It is usual to continue administration of a remedy only until some improvement is noted. Low potencies – where the substance has not been diluted to any great degree – have a relatively short-lasting effect; medium potencies have a wider influence; high potencies are more fundamental and can even be effectual some time after they have been discontinued. High potencies should be prescribed by a doctor only; for self-help it is advisable to use lower potencies. Frequency is important – every three or four hours until improvement; if there is no change after twenty-four hours, the choice of remedy is usually incorrect.

HUMAN AURA

Studies by metaphysicians have shown that there is a coloured rim surrounding the human body, known as the aura, and that the aura is a fact and not an illusionary effect seen by clairvoyants and those with extrasensory perception. It can now be explained in terms of energy, and it is becoming more apparent that all living things emanate a number of forms of energy. Think, for example, of the light around some deep-sea fish, fireflies and glow-worms.

Advanced technology has produced instruments which make it possible to scan the normal, non-energized aura. Earlier methods included ways of stepping up aural energy, intensifying it several times in order to see it. This often led to distortion. Now, by using methods to sensitize the human eye to the near ultraviolet light waves of the aura, it can now be viewed at its normal energy level.

It appears as a relatively bright bluish-grey mist about a centimetre deep outlining the skin – entirely surrounding it, including all the intricate ins and outs of the body form such as finger separations. Between the skin and the mist is a narrow dark space. Further out is a less precise circle of energy.

The characteristic aurae for different health patterns have been observed and established; variation in striations (rays of light that appear as bundles) of the inner aura indicate illness, and so aid medical diagnosis. (Mental states also affect the quality and intensity of the aura.) Physical disorders can be anticipated as far ahead as six weeks, as they are invariably preceded by a lessening and darkening of the aura over the area in question. Breaks in light over the skin surface specifically indicate a let-down in some function; for example, an arthritic joint will give off bright rays of light, interspaced with dark strips, at a right angle to the affected joint.

The bio-energetic aspects of the human aura are undergoing further exploration for its diagnostic value and for the light it throws on our understanding of life processes.

MUSIC THERAPY

It is well-known that music can relax and provide emotional refreshment; it can restore the mind, it can be a means of releasing pent-up energy and tension. However, its therapeutic powers can go further, and when presented within certain channels, music can be employed as a pleasant natural aid to some health conditions, related to both the physiological and psychological sides of medicine.

Music therapy works through the four elements contained in any sound: pitch, duration, tone and volume. There are two techniques – receptive and active – but both aim at re-establishing communication which has broken down due to illness or handicap: in the paralysed, the geriatric, the mentally disturbed, the spastic and the subnormal who have never related normally to the world.

At the receptive level, the patient listens; the music will influence mood and behaviour. The choice, of course, is the vital issue, and it has been shown that the music should relate to and reflect the state of mind at that time. Persuasion through opposites does not usually work; soft music is not soothing to an agitated mind, nor can brisk, happy music lessen depression. Initially the music must be on the same 'wavelength' as the emotions, and then can be gradually changed in a positive direction. This receptive technique can be used in psychiatric treatment, when music inspires confidence and can lead to the expression of buried emotions.

In an active way, a patient can be involved in making music, singing or playing. This is a social art, and music therapy of this type can be one of the best roads to rehabilitation within a group, as it forces communication, unity and discipline; it provides a common interest, a common goal, a basis for giving and taking.

Another interesting aspect of music therapy is in relation to asthmatic cases. If child sufferers are encouraged to take up wind instruments, the capacity of the lungs is increased and pulmonary health improved.

OSTEOPATHY

The name of this therapy is misleading, as osteopathy implies bone disorders; in practice it is a means of helping varied disorders connected with the circulatory system within the skeletal frame, and its implications can be far-reaching.

Osteopathy originated in America just over a hundred years ago; the founder was Dr Andrew Taylor Still. It is applicable to all age groups, though it is particularly valid for elderly people's troubles, women's disorders and problems of growth and development in children. It is often impossible to cure older people because of the extent of a chronic ailment, but osteopathy may help to keep them reasonably pain-free and functioning during their last years. Osteopathy is not a substitute for medicine or surgery, but it can be an effective alternative for structural problems in the musculo-skeletal system, low back pain and sciatica, muscular and ligament defects, tightened bands of connective tissue, and headaches of physical origin. It can also be helpful in certain nervous disorders that lead to migraine and reflex headaches, asthma, heart problems and ulcers.

A basic principle of osteopathy is that disease stems from malfunction of the circulatory system, primarily in the spinal area. The free flow of blood is essential for health, together with a smooth functioning of the lymphatic system. These processes can be hindered by any deviation from normality in bones, joints and soft tissues. Such abnormalities are called lesions and can be caused by falls, sprains, strains, blows, bad posture, bad diet or tension.

The art of the osteopath is to manipulate and massage lesions back to normality. This is not necessarily confined to the spinal column, though this is the primary focus; the pelvis, the feet, the chest wall or various joints may need attention. Treatment is preceded by a consultation and a manual examination, supported by the diagnostic methods of conventional medicine; areas of the body are touched to assess the rate, heat and quality of blood palpitating beneath them; X-rays are important. While using specific techniques, the treatment stresses integration of the whole body; case histories are detailed, and auxiliary alternative methods may be employed.

A session with a practitioner usually lasts about half an hour. The length of treatment depends on the condition, age and overall health. Weekly treatments over several months are the norm, though sometimes a problem will clear up after only a few manipulations. It is not often that treatment extends longer than a year.

RADIETHESIA AND RADIONICS

Radiethesia is sensitivity to radiations; it is an ancient art practised by skilled men through the ages, certainly as far back as the Egyptians 4,000 years ago. The first instruments were dowsers' twigs, divining rods and the pendulum. Now advanced technology has developed instruments that make use of certain human faculties that function in the realm of the mind – assuming that the human mind is a specialized form of computer. This modern technique is known as radionics and, using a hair or blood specimen of the patient, patterns of non-physical energy can be traced to identify the cause of an illness and recommend remedial treatment. The patient does not have to be present. Another point: most equipment, whether the basic tools of radiethesia such as the hazel fork, the simple pendulum and the black box, or the more sophisticated instruments used for radionics, will work for 90 per cent of people and for 100 per cent of psychics. It is basically a mind process; advanced neometaphysical practitioners suggest that with a little more psychological probing our mental powers could control our physical health.

Radionics appears to be mysterious because we have only just begun to rediscover the natural phenomena, laws and processes which can explain it. Science considered for many years that the intrinsic elements of the universe were energy and matter, but now it is emerging that matter itself is actually crystallized energy. The ultimate constituents of creation are energy and mind. This makes radionics plausible, as the cosmos is seen as a united force in which no part is completely separate from another – an immensely complex network of interlocking and interacting energies that manifest themselves in many ways and forms. Physical energies – electrical, nuclear and gravitational – are involved, but the more elusive non-physical energy fields are believed to be much more important. These include, for example, the Hindu *prana*, the Chinese *ch'i*, the *yin* and *yang* forces, the life force of western interpretations.

It is at the non-physical level that radionics makes its analysis and recommends treatments. It is refined radiethesia. The sample hair or drop of blood is not analysed but serves as a tuning link between the patient and practitioner. It is advisable for the practitioner to see the patient before treatment, but it is not essential.

The instruments used in radionics are highly complicated; they are manipulated by dials and figures which are associated with various parts of the body, recording and calculating the feedback. With knowledge of the patient's medical history, the symptoms can be analysed, the complaint diagnosed and treatment suggested. It is not simply a question of telepathy or extrasensory perception, but of mental command of energy fields in relation to physical forms. In a simple ailment, diagnosis and prescription may take twenty minutes; more complicated illnesses could take hours.

Patients are often advised to seek medication through orthodox or alternative medical practitioners, or warned that surgery may be necessary.

REFLEXOLOGY

A treatment based on the principle that there is a direct reflex action between the nerve endings on the soles of the feet and the various organs of the body. It is a very specialized form of compressed massage and pressure. Also known as 'zone therapy', it is of Chinese origin and was brought to the western world about eighty years ago by an American doctor, William H. FitzGerald. It was popularized in the 1930s by a masseuse, Eunice Ingham, whose method – the Ingham Reflex Method of Compression Massage – is still used today.

The soles and parts of the upper foot make up a complete chart of the body's vital organs and functions – a sort of condensed body map or guide. Diagnostically, all parts of the body have a reflex point on the feet. By sensitively feeling the feet, one at a time, an experienced practitioner can detect a disorder by changes in texture under the surface of the skin. Usually there is a crystal-like deposit, sometimes a shallow depression. The therapist applies gentle thumb and finger pressure to the point; the patient may feel pain, a sensation of having a needle or glass stuck in the foot; extremely sensitive people may even feel pain in the organ itself. The more extreme the reaction, the more serious the disorder. No two patients are alike in reaction; one may feel very cold, another may undergo emotional distress.

Reflexology can be used for diagnosis, as a preventive measure and as a treatment. During treatment, pressure is continued evenly on the appropriate point and at the same time a clockwise rotating massage is applied. As the pain at the pressure point decreases, the health of the organ improves – sometimes, it is claimed, quite dramatically. Treatments last about twenty minutes; a second treatment is recommended after a few days. If pain remains, treatment is continued, but rarely more than once or twice a week.

It particularly helps conditions involving congestion: sinus problems, migraine, stimulation of pancreas and liver; it is effective for constipation and kidney disorders – it has been known to stimulate the passing of very small gravel stones and even kidney stones. Toxic elements that hinder organic function and block the natural flow of energy may be successfully dispersed. Sometimes treatment builds up the body's own healing forces; in this respect it is often aided by other natural therapies.

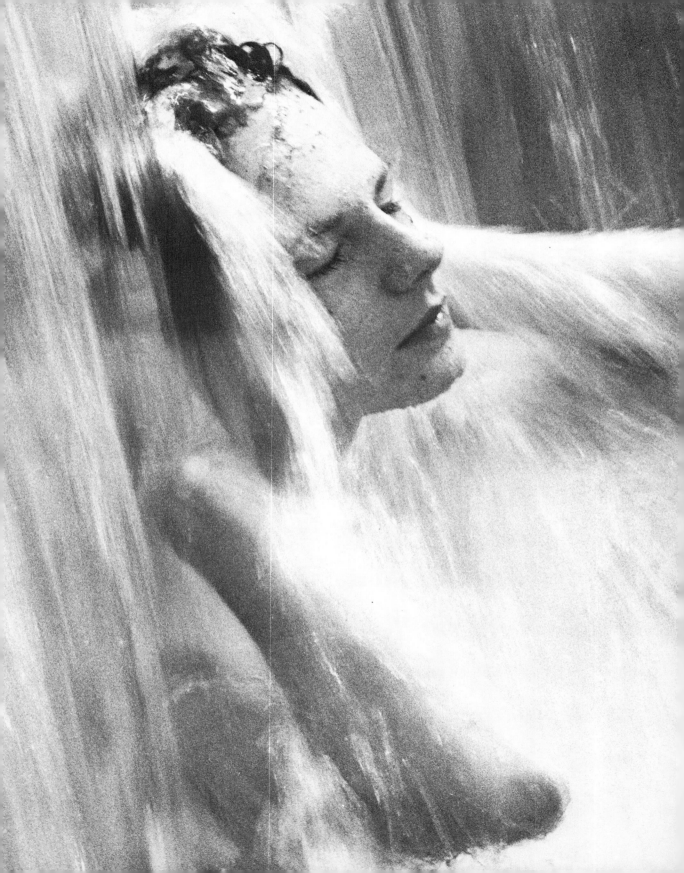

6

HEALTH SPAS

Not all health spas are alike. They basically fall into three categories. First, there are the traditional ones, with cures centering on the value of certain waters and with an emphasis on hydrotherapy. They treat specific physical or nervous problems. America has many areas with therapeutic waters, and institutions have developed around them. Unfortunately, they are not very well known. In Europe 'taking the waters' has been a medical tradition for centuries. Entire towns turn themselves into one big healing emporium. It is usual to stay in a hotel, where a doctor is recommended and special provision is made for dietary régimes. Treatment facilities are available either on the hotel premises or in near-by establishments and all the therapies are given under medical supervision. You can thus combine a holiday and a cure. Except for specific treatments, you are free to organize your own activities. Most European spas offer cultural programmes, sightseeing and, invariably, a casino. In America, musical and theatrical entertainment are popular additions. Nearly all spas have in-patient sanatoria for serious cases.

Second are the nature-cure clinics, where naturopathic doctors practise their belief that the body has to build up its own resistance to disease. Surgery and synthetic drugs are considered last resorts – natural remedies are used with emphasis on fasting, nutrition and herbal treatments. Hydrotherapy is used, in addition to many of the natural therapeutics mentioned in the previous chapter. The irony is that these clinics frequently help patients who have been abandoned by orthodox practitioners. Nature-cure clinics are often in the vicinity of natural spas.

Third, there is the health resort – a cross between a clinic and a high-class hotel. The entire day is scheduled, a diet is provided, and you are under constant supervision to ensure that you do not stray from the programme. It is rather like an adult camp and perfect for those who lack the will-power, concentration, and self-discipline to keep their bodies in top condition – and at the right weight. These health spas plan for each individual a programme that revitalizes the system, adds or reduces weight, tones up body muscles, and helps counteract stress and tension. However, a most important feature is re-education – learning new health rules of nutrition and general body care, so that you go away not only looking and feeling better, but equipped with the knowledge of how to stay that way and how to be aware of the body's needs and changes.

MINERAL WATER SPAS

The chief minerals in spa water are sodium, calcium, magnesium, carbon and sulphur. Many springs are radioactive although not to the point of being dangerous unless taken daily over many years. The waters may be drunk or the skin may be exposed to them. Each spa has its own rules as to amounts, which of course depend upon the content. Taken internally, the water can directly influence the digestive organs, then go through the liver into the blood circulation and finally be eliminated through the kidneys. In this way the water introduces various salts and minerals to all areas of the body in a naturally balanced composition. Externally, mineral waters stimulate the skin, improving circulation and toning muscles. Hydrotherapy (see Environment, pages 60–66) also helps the skin adapt to changes of heat and cold – inefficiency in this can lead to many diseases. The therapeutic value of hydrotherapy is said to be improved in specific cases when certain substances are present:

Iodine: Good for high blood pressure, various eye diseases, chronic inflammation of the female organs, circulatory problems.

Iron: Helps anaemia.

Sulphur: Aids rheumatic conditions, metabolic disorders and skin diseases.

Sodium chloride: Significant in the correction of women's diseases, circulation and the adjustment of functional disorders.

Radon: Eases pain, helps correct imbalance of the endocrine glands, reduces nerve inflammation.

Glauber's salt (sodium sulphate): Helps obesity, diabetes and gout; in particular encourages the production of bile and its entry into the intestines, consequently reviving the elasticity of the gall bladder.

Acidulous waters: An aid for the heart muscles and circulation, particularly in cases where these are weak due to alcohol and smoking; also recommended for diseases of the respiratory tract and urological disorders.

Natural spa resorts are very organized when it comes to information on their facilities – the composition of the waters, the medical indications, and accommodations. In the U.S.A. you can write to the chamber of commerce of the particular town for all details. For information about the European spas, write to the individual National Tourist Boards (mostly located in New York City) and ask for full information. Following is a summary of what you can expect at some of the most significant areas.

UNITED STATES

California is particularly blessed with natural health resources, but then it is a volcanic region. Palm Springs Spa makes good use of its mineral waters, but a flourishing area is twelve miles north where there are literally hundreds of hot mineral springs at Desert Hot Springs. These waters have been used by nomadic Indians for countless centuries as a source of healing. Apart from private facilities, there are several public mineral swimming pools. Another mecca for ancient tribes was Murietta Hot Springs, which at more than 1,300 feet above sea level has a most agreeable and even climate all year round. It is known particularly for its help in arthritic and rheumatic ailments. Another important centre for arthritis is Jacumba Hot Springs, east of San Diego. North east of San Francisco are the Calistoga Spas, where natural sulphur is directed into pools and steam cabinets and a special feature is a steam mud bath deriving from volcanic ash.

Sulphur in the form of steam as well as permeating the mud is also found at Holmes Sulphur Spring Bath, Sulphur Springs, Arkansas. Treatments for arthritis, locomotor injuries, and nervous disorders are given at Hot Springs National Park, Little Rock, Arkansas. In Florida – and remember Ponce de Leon thought he had found the fountain of youth there – Sarasota is probably the most renowned natural health resort. There is also the Carlsbad Spa, Hollywood, and Safety Harbor Spa, Safety Harbor. Even in the cooler climes therapeutic waters can be found: Saratoga Springs has had a good reputation for years, so has Alden Mineral Springs – both in New York

State. Sulphur is considered particularly curative – you'll find it in White Sulphur Spring, West Virginia, and in Sulphur, Oklahoma.

EUROPE

Spas on the Continent are booming. This is because they have the backing of the medical profession. They offer the traditional mixture of medicinal waters, used internally or externally, rest and relaxation. There is also a growing feeling amongst the public that naturopathic practitioners have a lot to offer and that the body should be given the opportunity to try to assimilate and to test the power of nature.

Austria

There are about one hundred spas, controlled by government regulations, including twenty with traditional Kniepp hydrotherapy (see Environment, page 62). One of the largest and most important is the Salzburg Therapeutic Centre, where all hydrotherapy methods are included. Others of note are Bad Gastein-Boeckstein, Bad Hall, Bad Haering and Bad Schoenau. Treatments used include baths with thermal, sulphur, iodine and radon waters; peat and mud baths; carbonic acid gas baths.

Czechoslovakia

There are about a hundred well-equipped health resorts and an equal number of thermal and mineral springs. The best known of these are Carlsbad (now Karlovy Vary) and Marienbad (or Marianské Lazne). At Carlsbad, those suffering from digestive, liver and metabolic diseases, as well as obesity, are treated. It has forty different hot mineral springs, producing about 440,000 gallons (2 million litres) of medicinal waters per day at a temperature of 161°F (71·7°C). Most visitors stay for an average of three or four weeks: a slow healing process is stressed, with walking and drinking the waters three times a day an important ritual. Marienbad has thirty-nine springs with emphasis on radon and carbon-dioxide hydrotherapies, including steam inhalation to aid respiratory problems.

France

With 1,200 mineral springs it is well endowed in medical water resources.

All spas are very much under public supervision, while in the medical field balneology is considered very important, with chairs in many universities. Vichy is the most significant centre due to the high sodium bicarbonate content of its waters. It is very good for liver complaints – often giving long-lasting results for disorders of the alimentary canal and digestion, for diabetes, gout and gallstones. Aix-les-Bains in the French Alps is renowned for the treatment of all kinds of rheumatic complaints, neuralgia, after-effects of fractures and wounds and infantile paralysis. Contrexéville has strong mineral springs reputedly excellent for gout, obesity and arthritis. At La Bourboule (Puy-de-Dôme) the waters are rich in radioactive elements that can help ear, nose and throat ailments and are also good for bronchitis, sinusitis, allergies and skin complaints. There are many thalassotherapy centres in France, where the sea water and marine climate are used for therapeutic purposes. The same bathing techniques are employed as for inland areas, and the sea water is heated to the desired temperature. Mud baths and baths containing seaweed are invariably part of the treatment. Thalassotherapy is said to help particularly rheumatism, painful spinal problems, tension, stress and depression.

Germany

In West Germany, spas go hand in hand with regular medical practices to such an extent that spa therapy is prescribed and covered financially by the social services. This means that the German spas are medically extremely efficient, but often difficult to get into. There are between 250 and 300 and one for almost every ailment. The best known on an international level include Bad Nauheim, where heart and circulatory problems are treated; the waters, rich in carbonic acid, also help alleviate rheumatic pain and improve the mobility of the joints. Bad Homburg is also a centre for the treatment of heart problems and metabolic diseases, including gout and obesity. Perhaps the most famous – and certainly the most elegant – is Baden-Baden situated on the rim of the Black Forest; its brine water, sulphur springs, mud and peat are helpful for general rejuvenation and for arthritic complaints in particular. Others of note are Wiesbaden, Bad Pyrmont and Aachen (Aix-la-Chapelle).

Great Britain

In Great Britain the natural mineral spas have been sadly neglected over the last fifty years, despite the fact that the waters are as beneficial as those on the Continent. There is, however, a restoration programme under way sponsored by national organizations. At the moment the best include Bath – Britain's oldest spa dating from about 800 B.C. Half a million gallons of mineral water rise daily in thermal springs. It is helpful in the treatment of all rheumatic diseases, gout, certain conditions of high blood pressure and metabolic disorders. Buxton is another spa in use since Roman times and still flourishing today. Thermal waters are used to treat rheumatic diseases and locomotor disorders. Droitwich has one of the most concentrated natural salt waters in the world, ten times saltier than normal sea water and great for rheumatism.

Italy

Apart from the many mineral waters, the mud-bath treatment is a speciality of Italian spas. Abano, together with the Montegrotto Spa, is the most important mud therapy centre in Europe. The mud, of volcanic origin, is the main treatment and is matured in special tanks. Its use is primarily indicated for chronic diseases of the locomotor system (anything to do with movement) and for abdominal inflammation following gynaecological disorders. At Salsomaggiore, the iodine waters are used for gynaecological conditions and treatment also includes mud baths. Montecatini is possibly the best-known spa in Italy; treatment is given for liver and bile duct disorders, diseases of the digestive system and urinary tract problems. Again, mud baths are an integral part of the therapy. At Ischia, an island off the coast near Naples, recuperative waters are found in an idyllic setting. They are alkaline, containing sodium chloride and bicarbonates; they are also highly radioactive. The great variety and complexity of the biological actions of the waters offer wide therapeutic possibilities. They are good for chronic arthropathy after injury, for diseases of the peripheral nervous system, for gynaecological disorders resulting from hormone disturbances or inflammation of the pelvic organs and for metabolic diseases including gout and obesity. Treatments include both hydropathic and mud baths.

Switzerland

The climate and altitude of certain resorts is considered to be as important as the waters, sometimes more so. Swiss health centres are suitable for convalescence, disturbances of old age, tension, stress and disorders of the pulmonary and respiratory tracts. St Moritz has the highest medicinal springs in Switzerland and the highest content of carbonic acid and iron of any waters in Europe. The air is dry and free from allergies. It is good for the heart and circulation, gynaecological disorders and tropical diseases. Disentis has an acidulous chalybeate spring that is the most highly radioactive one in the area; it is used primarily in the treatment of circulatory problems and high blood pressure. Bad Ragaz has an abundant spring rising to 99°F (37·2°C), which is good for rheumatism, paralysis, lesions of vertebral discs and diseases of the veins. Scuoi, Tarasp and Vulpera are famous for their mineral springs, which yield Glauber's salt: they are recommended for liver and bile complaints, gall stones, stomach and intestinal disorders, constipation, obesity and diabetes.

NATURE-CURE CLINICS

Establishments vary in what they have to offer. Common to all, though, is the basic principle that food is your best medicine. It is said to cause or cure disease depending on its origin, composition, and preparation. A fresh vegetarian régime is the normal fare. Many clinics stress the importance of a fast, which means you sip lemon tea for a minimum of three days, or you may be restricted to only fruit or vegetable juices. The importance of exercise is also stressed as being essential to health. Even if it is only walking or gentle swimming (as opposed to calisthenics) exercise improves circulation, helps break-up fat deposits, and encourages elimination. For patients who require special attention to certain organs, there are always programmed remedial exercises. Colonic irrigation is regarded as a necessity in most clinics. Osteopathic and chiropractic treatments are used for spinal, joint and muscle problems. Alcohol and smoking are not allowed. The length of stay depends upon the seriousness of the illness. Here is a selection of some of the leading international nature-cure clinics. Brochures are available giving full details on accommodation, treatment facilities and prices.

UNITED STATES

Florida Spa,
Orlando, Florida

Hidden Valley Health Ranch,
Escondido, California

Meadowlark Spa,
26126 Fairview Ave,
Hemet, California

Pritikin Clinic,
Santa Barbara, California

Shangri-La,
Bonita Springs, Florida

Villa Vegetariana,
P.O. Box 1228,
Cuernavaca, Mexico

Vita Dell Spa,
13495 Palm Drive,
Desert Hot Springs, California

FRANCE

Thalassotherapy Institute,
Quiberon, Brittany

GERMANY

Buchinger-Klinik am Bodensee,
Uberlingen

GREAT BRITAIN

Enton Hall,
near Godalming, Surrey

Forest Mere Health Hydro,
Liphook, Hampshire

Shrubland Hall Health Clinic,
Coddenham, near Ipswich, Suffolk

Tyringham Naturopathic Clinic,
Newport Pagnell, Buckinghamshire

SPAIN

Clinica Buchinger Marbella,
Apartado 68,
Marbella, Malaga

SWITZERLAND

Bircher-Benner Clinic,
Zürich

HEALTH RESORTS

The aim of this type of spa – apart from the obvious visible benefits – is to give you a new incentive to maintain health and body shape. The length of stay should not be less than five days, and most resorts insist on a minimum of a week, usually beginning on Sunday. Accommodations are often luxurious. Most provide facilities such as swimming pools, solariums, gardens, tennis courts, and indoor activities, and have access to golf courses and riding stables. On arrival, assuming you have no specific health problems, the doctor will give you a general health check, taking details of past medical history. You will be weighed, and if you need to lose weight, a target figure will be set. A personal programme is compiled – a day might go something like this: 7.30, breakfast; 8.30, exercises; 9.30, water or steam treatments; 10.30, massage; 11.00, special treatment (beauty or other-wise); 12.00, water exercise; 1.00, lunch; 2.00, special treatment; 3.00, gymnastics; 4.00, yoga instruction; 5.00, rest or beauty treatments; 6.30, dinner; 8.00, evening activity. Programmes are usually tightly organized and vary each day according to progress and reaction to the various treatments and therapies. There are hours set aside for those who like walking, jogging or sports. Days pass constructively and pleasantly. A work-out week at a spa could be your best vacation; some are more gruelling than others, some more pampering. With all there's the comforting thought that you will go home pounds lighter and considerably more fit. Below are listed the leading health resorts in America with a few details on atmosphere, policy, and programmes, plus a listing of the more important European resorts.

UNITED STATES

American Fitness Institute,
P.O. Box 2615,
Park City, Utah

Set in a woody mountain area at an altitude of 7,200 feet, the emphasis is on diet re-education, through teaching you how to change bad eating habits. Weight control – through the mind and through the body – is very definitely the main preoccupation. In the diet, calorie counting is not important, it's the type of food that is stressed: a high complex-carbohydrate diet, geared for high energy. Meals are buffet style, and there are campfire cook-outs. Aerobics are favoured for exercise, graded according to capacity. There are cooking classes for low-calorie eating.

Canyon Ranch Vacation/Fitness Resort,
8600 East Rockcliff Road,
Tuscon, Arizona

This is a dry, desert climate in the foothills of the Catalina Mountains. The resort puts the accent on relaxation and provides an unpressured pro-gramme that mixes vacation activities with exercise and treatments.

The Ashram,
Calabasas,
California

A very small intimate retreat, where physical exhaustion is considered very healthy, run by the Swedish fitness expert Anne-Marie Bennstrom. This is a resort for the hardy – expect no pampering here. Intensive physical activity is the daily rule. The diet is strictly two alternatives: entirely raw – fruits, vegetables, seeds, berries, etc. – or a total fast offering three days of fresh fruit juices alternated with three days of herb teas and water. Weight loss is considered incidental in comparison to health improvement, but on such a regimen can be between 8 to 10 pounds a week.

World of Palm-Aire,
Palm-Aire Drive North,
Pompano Beach, Florida

This is really a luxury resort with four hotels located on 2,400 acres between West Palm Beach and Miami. It is tropical, it has a holiday air about it, and under the joint directorship of Lisa Dobloug and Jacques Piguet it has become one of the most popular spas in the country. They do not believe in martyrdom even in the interest of body health and beauty. Nevertheless special emphasis is on correct breathing, posture, cardiovascular fitness, and relaxation. Treatment runs the full gamut expected in such spas; diet ranges from 600 to 1,000 calories daily – three meals with a choice of fish, fowl, vegetables, fruit, herbal teas. Lots goes on after hours along the Gold Coast, but beware of temptation to stray from those sensible diet plans – and that includes no drinking.

EUROPE

In Europe the health resort is not so common as it is in the United States because the grand hotels in the spa towns offer similar facilities, although not in a controlled environment. Self-restraint is not easy, particularly when overseas, so here are the best places to go for constant supervision and definite rules about the rest of the world being out of bounds.

Opposite: Khu Khan, 1978
Overleaf left: Mike Reinhardt, 1974
Overleaf right: Hans Seurer, 1972

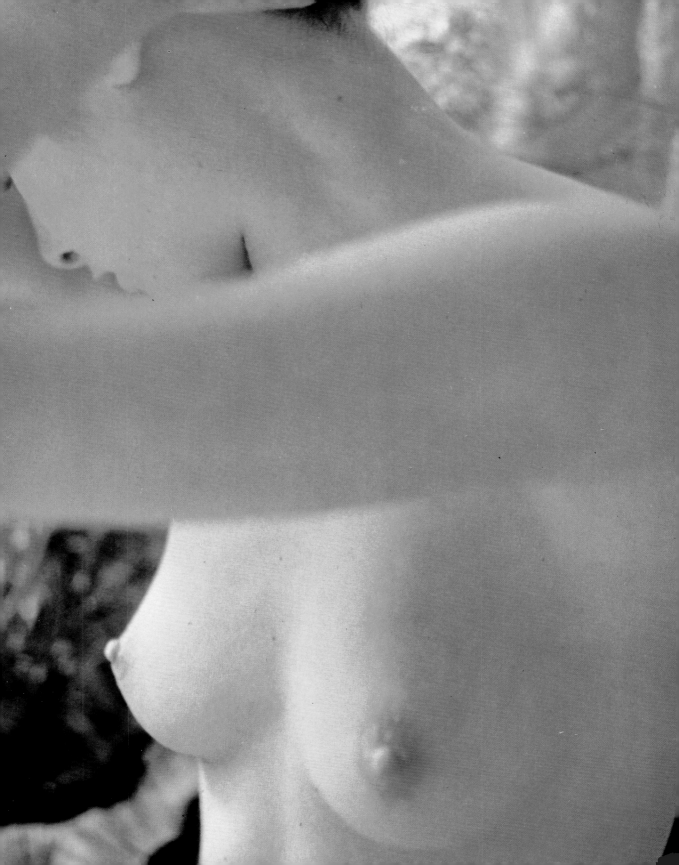

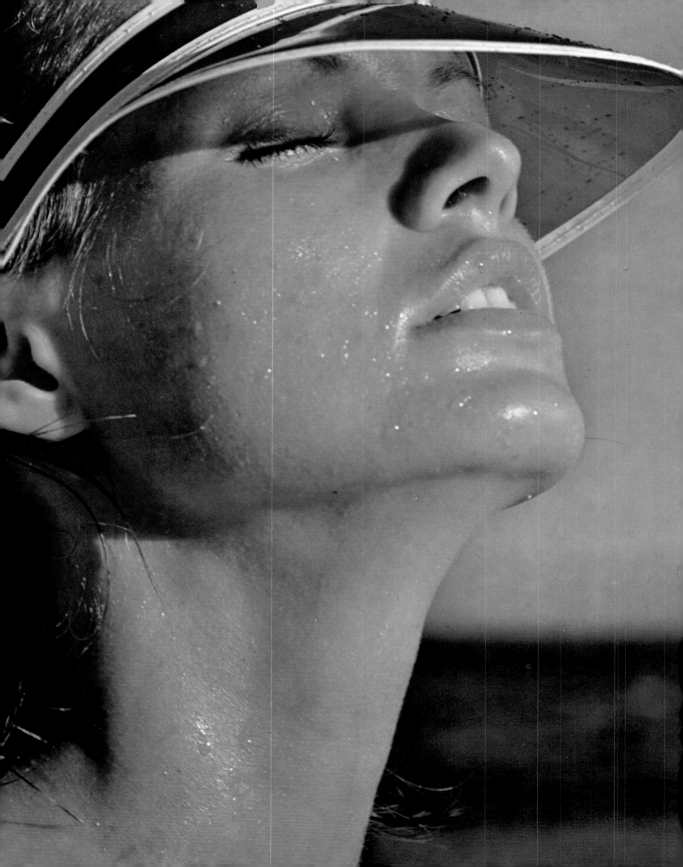

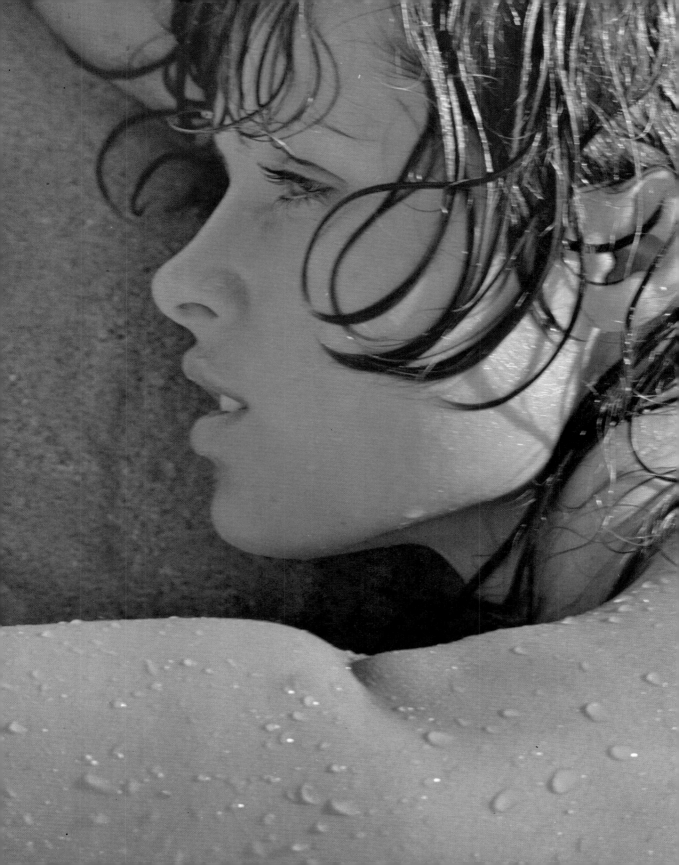

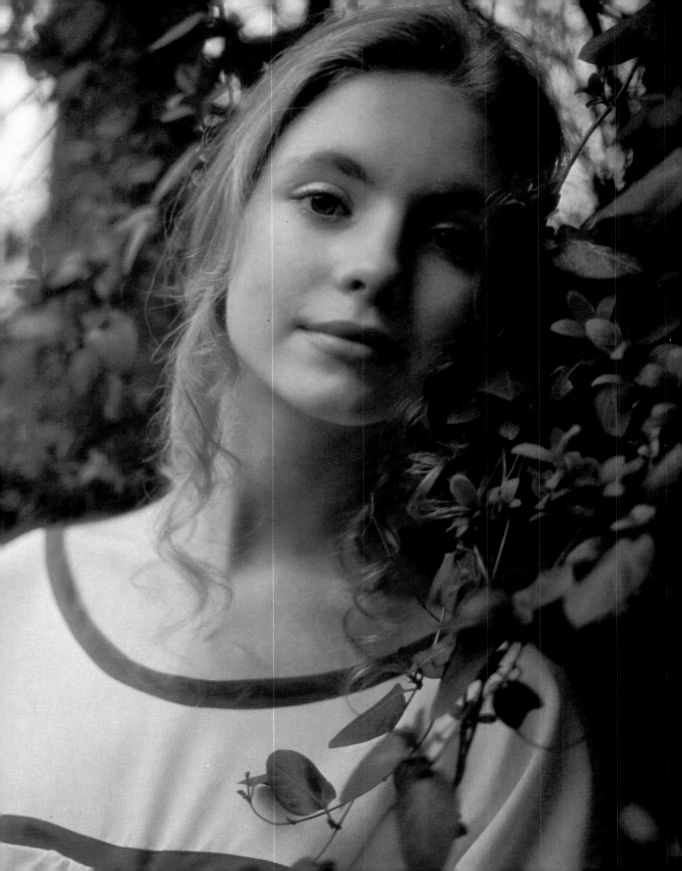

France

La Maison des Prés et des Sources d'Eugénie,
Eugénie-les-Bains

Great Britain

Champneys Health Resort,
Tring, Hertfordshire

Chevin Hall Health and Beauty Hotel,
Otley, Yorkshire

Grayshott Hall Health Centre,
Grayshott, near Hindhead, Surrey

Henlow Grange Beauty Farm,
Henlow, Bedfordshire

The Imperial Relaxation Centre,
Imperial Hotel,
Torquay, Devonshire

Stobo Castle Health and Beauty Spa,
Peeblesshire, Scotland

Spain

Brisamer,
Fuente del Perro

Incosol,
Marbella

Switzerland

Belmilon,
Grand Hôtel Beau Rivage,
Interlaken

Calories are controlled here (800 to 850 a day) and portion size is considered important. Meals are served in a main dining room.

Ilona of Hungary,
3201 East Second Avenue,
Denver, Colorado

Skin perfection is the aim here with the emphasis on head to toe skin and beauty-care; the guiding principle is that improving the outside also improves what's within. Skin analysis is given and treatment established accordingly – with such European specialties as aromatherapy, herbal wraps, and lymph drainage. Weight loss here is a gradual thing in the interests of the look of the skin, its elasticity, its need to shrink slowly for good lasting effects. Diet includes lean meat, vegetables, and fruits.

New Life Health Spa at Liftline Lodge,
Stratton Mount,
Vermont

A small personalized spa that functions only in the summer. Yoga is the focal point – a mind and body recharge programme through Eastern philosophy, including meditation. Diet is a personalized plan of no more than 800 calories a day – all low sodium foods, chicken, fish, or vegetarian.

Rancho La Puerta,
Tecate, Baja California

Founded forty years ago by Deborah and Edmond Bordeaux Szekely, Rancho La Puerta was the harbinger of all health resorts in America, the first to introduce the concept of naturally healthful eating and living that other spas preach today. Ms Szekely is also the director of the Golden Door in Escondido, California – one of the most luxurious spas anywhere. The idea at Rancho La Puerta – as it was right from the very beginning – is that fitness is a way of life, a matter of enlightened thinking and not just physical well being. The programme shows you how you can incorporate regular daily exercise (outdoor and indoor activity) and a properly balanced natural diet into your life-style. Diet on the ranch is primarily lacto-ovo vegetarian, with fish dishes twice a week; important is a juice-only diet day. Activity is grouped under 'moderate' or 'vigorous'. A voluntary schedule involves a 6.30 a.m. mountain hike or moderate walk or wake-up exercises.

WATER

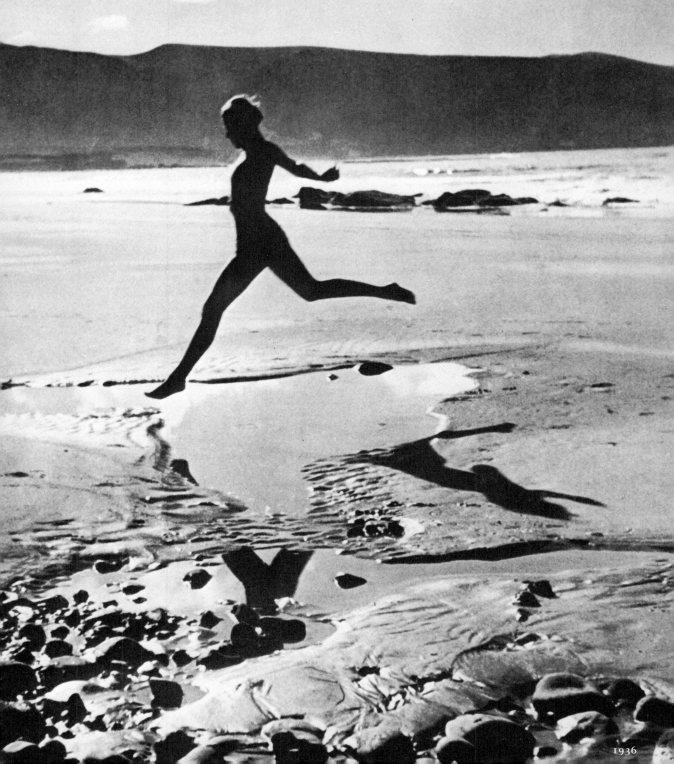

1936

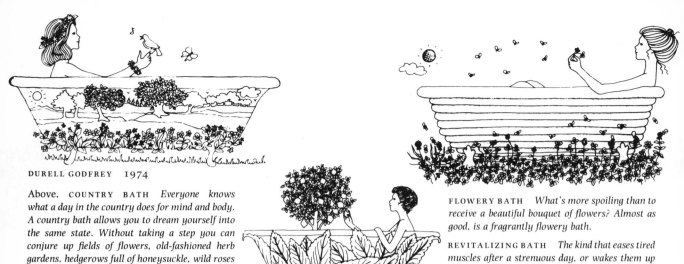

DURELL GODFREY 1974

Above, COUNTRY BATH *Everyone knows what a day in the country does for mind and body. A country bath allows you to dream yourself into the same state. Without taking a step you can conjure up fields of flowers, old-fashioned herb gardens, hedgerows full of honeysuckle, wild roses and moss.*

FLOWERY BATH *What's more spoiling than to receive a beautiful bouquet of flowers? Almost as good, is a fragrantly flowery bath.*

REVITALIZING BATH *The kind that eases tired muscles after a strenuous day, or wakes them up the morning after the night before – gives body and mind a new lease of life for the next few hours.*

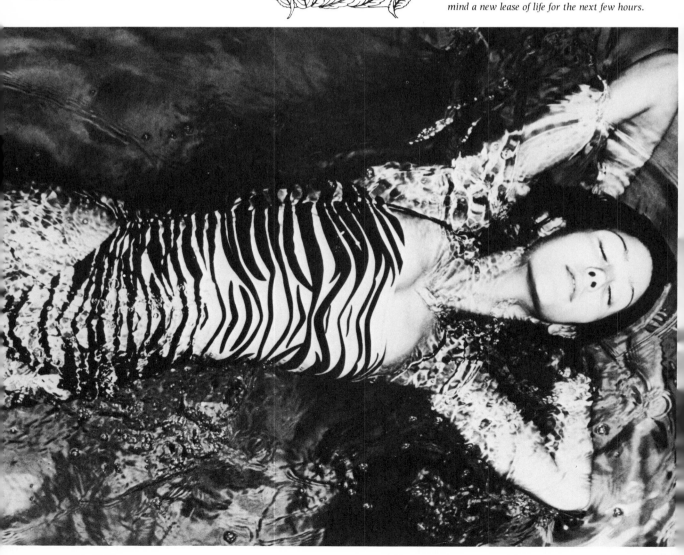

JOHN SWANNELL 1978

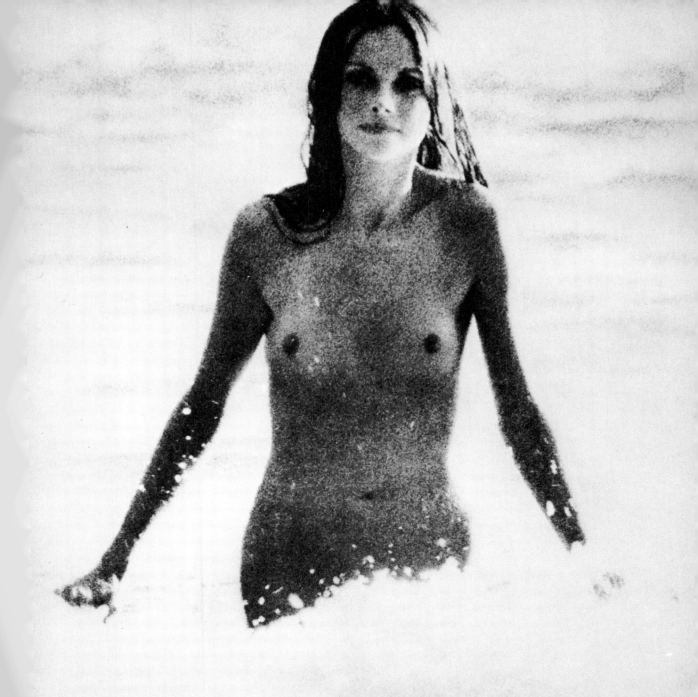

DAVID BAILEY 1970

PART II POWER OF PLANTS

LESTER BOOKBINDER

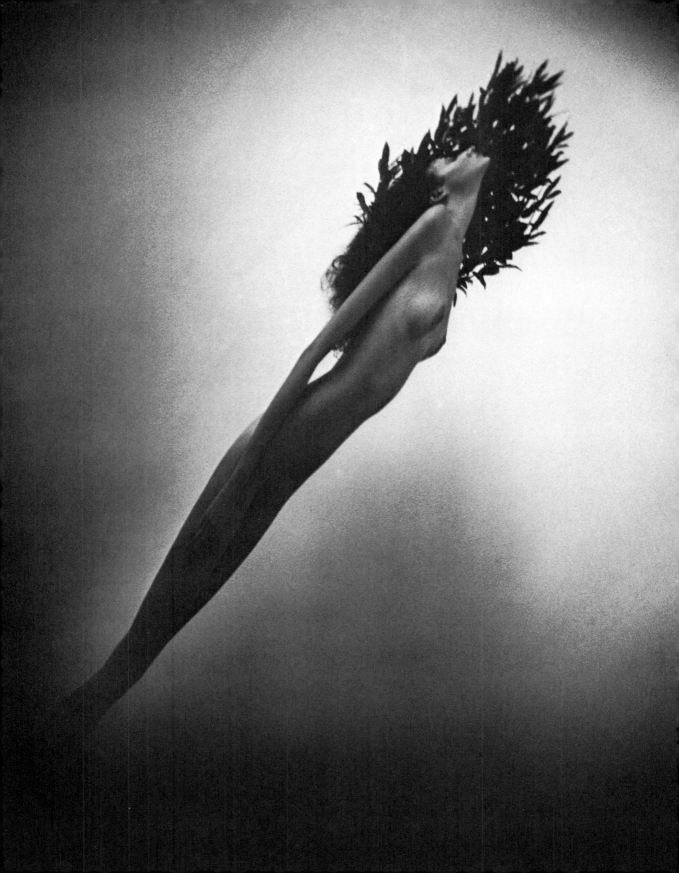

T he resurgence of interest in the healing power of plants is due in part to a growing anxiety about the widespread use of drugs and the possibility of serious side-effects. There is also an increasing awareness that our health, and particularly the prevention of illness, is our personal responsibility.

The question is: to what extent can sickness be prevented or cured by foods and herbal remedies? There is no absolute answer, though many research projects are currently under way; hitherto it has been the individual doctor or the small clinic that has provided constructive information. There are two opposing camps – those who firmly believe in plant power, and the more orthodox who dismiss it.

The claims concerning the healing qualities of plants are widespread and well-founded. Even though herbal remedies fell from general favour in the nineteenth century, they continued to be used in isolated country areas. And, in fact, a quarter of pharmaceutical remedies used today are of plant origin. A glance through a pharmacopoeia which lists all drugs reveals, for example, that hawthorn helps reduce blood pressure, hazelwort is used for headaches and comfrey as an application to wounds, broken bones and ulcers.

Some herbal remedies have been in use for as long as four thousand years, such as the Chinese fir which is used in the treatment of asthma and bronchitis. Not until 1878 was it discovered that its juice contains the alkaloid ephedrine which is much used in the treatment of pulmonary disorders today. This is but one instance of proven efficacy; and there are so many that botanists and chemists are now taking a new look at the plants which have traditionally been used for healing. This is a branch of medicine known as pharmacognosy.

A pharmacognostist deals with the past in the light of present knowledge. Herbal remedies were generally empirical – no one really knew how or why they worked and for generations little was understood about the mech- anisms and causes of disease. Today's task is to identify the bio-active elements and chemicals in the plants, isolate them for further studies and attempt chemical synthesis.

But to traditional practitioners of herbal medicine this seems like proving a point only to revert to the contemporary drug situation. They are not happy about synthetic chemical substitutes of specific molecules, arguing that the other ingredients in a plant either accelerate the active matter or act to prevent overdose or side-effects. They say that this complex mingling of protein, vitamins, enzymes, trace minerals and salts accounts for the lack of toxicity in plant remedies. Plants in their natural form work by increasing the body's own resistance to disease.

It is a basic tenet of herbalism that plants of one kind or another can not only treat a general disorder, but can also heal a particular organ or a particular part of an organ – this is one of the major differences between herbalism and folk medicine. It is also more sophisticated and precise; it uses a greater variety of plant materials in various forms and in carefully measured amounts, frequently in combination. The folk tradition commonly relies upon local plants, used singly.

Homoeopathy also employs herbs medicinally and there are about two thousand remedies that make up the homoeopathic pharmacopoeia. Their methods, however, are different: the plant extracts are highly potentized – diluted to an infinitesimal degree (see pages 79–81). Aromatherapy (see pages 140–42) employs the essential oils of a wide variety of plants; the unique Bach flower remedies (see pages 137–40) are potentized extracts that help the body by adjusting the emotional state. All these therapeutic systems have one thing in common: they formulate remedies from living vegetation.

Although many people would be better off if they knew more about the value of plants, herbal medicines should never be looked upon as a substitute for professional help. They can sensibly be used in conjunction with other forms of treatment and can be taken as strengtheners, preventatives and correctives for minor disturbances.

The terminology may seem confusing, as the word 'herb' implies different things to different people; to some it is a flavouring for food, to others a tea – and to these it comes as quite a surprise to find that certain vegetables, fruits and flowers are also referred to as 'herbs'. To the herbalist a herb is any plant that can aid the body, be it a bush, tree, flower or shrub. They are divided here into three groups according to their common categories and their use and preparation:

1. Vegetables and fruits – familiar varieties, eaten intact or as a juice; external applications.

2. Herbs and tisanes – well-known garden and wild plants, also foliage of vegetables and fruits, made into teas to drink or into poultices or lotions for surface problems.

3. Essences and flowers – extracts as oils or tinctures taken orally or applied externally.

The plants listed here have been selected from a long list on the basis of being the most well-known and readily available plants that together can supply most of the layman's needs. It is best to start with a few plants and become thoroughly familiar with their preparation and uses. The treatments given here are for maintenance, prevention and, to a limited extent, correction; self-medication is not advisable when persistent or serious conditions prevail – it is then essential to seek advice from a qualified practitioner in any of the botanical medical arts.

In general, awareness and practice of the following principles will fortify physical and mental balance. But remember that help through nature is a slow process; it is consistent use over a period of time that brings results. When you get into the habit of drinking herbal tea instead of coffee, of looking to raw juices for nourishment, of treating essences as more than a pleasant smell, then you are well on the way to keeping yourself healthy.

1
VEGETABLES AND FRUITS

Vegetables and fruits are the most accessible and certainly the simplest form of natural medicine. They are best eaten raw and are also effective when taken as a juice. Juices are, of course, easier to consume, and at times the only way to benefit therapeutically. For instance, it would be impossible for most people to eat sufficient raw cabbage to obtain the required amount for treatment of a gastric ulcer, whereas a pint or two of liquid is easily swallowed. An electric juice extractor is one of the best health investments.

The regular addition to a basic diet (see pages 13–16) of the following vegetables and fruits can strengthen the body and assist in prevention of metabolic breakdowns. Freshness is of paramount importance; vegetables and fruit begin to deteriorate as soon as they are gathered, though if eaten reasonably fresh the loss in value is slight. Cooking considerably reduces their power and that is why the raw vegetable or juice is always recommended for medicinal use. For general nutrition, cooking within certain principles is beneficial for body maintenance.

It is important to remember that natural aids do their job very slowly. Larger amounts do not necessarily mean faster results; regular controlled doses are more effective. It is impossible to eat too much of the whole vegetable or fruit: satiation would come first. The rule on juices is from 1 to 8 pints (2 to 16 cups) a day, but never more than is comfortable. See pages 108–115 for treatments for specific disorders.

External applications – as poultices or lotions – not only help surface conditions but often have the capacity to infuse skin layers and influence internal organs. A poultice of cooked pulp will help aches and pains, slow-healing wounds and inflammation of the eyelids. A poultice of raw grated apple will help the pain of a black eye.

APPLE

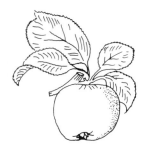

Traditionally the great health provider, both preventive and curative, it is particularly high in mineral salts (a larger quantity of phosphates than any other vegetable or fruit) and rich in vitamins, and in addition provides pectin, amino acids and natural sugars. Apples are best eaten before meals, first thing in the morning or last thing at night (they also encourage sleep). They help overcome liverishness, digestive disturbances and encourage flushing of the kidneys. Apple juice is good as a drink; on a curative basis take a minimum of a pint a day. (Unsweetened cider can be taken as an alternative.) Cider vinegar also retains the health-giving properties – 2 teaspoons in a glass of water, once or twice a day. Apples are prescribed for intestinal infections, mental and physical fatigue, demineralization, urine retention, rheumatism and gout; they are also recommended for coughs, hoarseness and pulmonary conditions. Some doctors advise apples to combat excess cholesterol in the blood.

Another alternative to the fresh juice drink is: 3 large unpeeled apples, sliced and covered with 5 cups cold water, add 2 teaspoons honey and boil for 15 minutes, strain, drink tepid. If taken to alleviate a fever, drink cold.

ARTICHOKE (GLOBE)

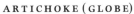

This contains therapeutically valuable oils which have a strong stabilizing effect on the human metabolism. It is particularly beneficial for the liver and acts as a diuretic for those suffering from water retention. It can protect against urea, cholesterol and arthritis. The juice can be pressed from the stem and leaves, but it is very bitter. To relieve rheumatism take 2 – 3 teaspoons before meals – the taste can be improved if mixed with a small glass of wine.

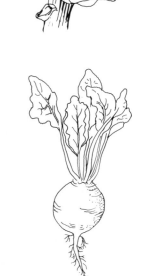

BEETS

The amino acids are good both in quality and quantity and naturopathic practitioners consider the juice to be one of the most therapeutic. It is effective in cases of general weakness and is used as a restorative during convalescence. The root contains about one tenth pure sugar, which provides energy. In France, interesting results have been obtained by treating malignant disease with huge quantities of the juice, 6–7 pints (3·5

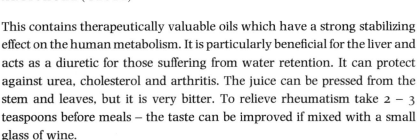

−4l.) a day; however, there is not yet enough medical evidence to substantiate findings. Beet juice combined with carrot and cucumber juices builds up the blood and is helpful in the treatment of kidney stones, gall bladder, liver and prostate troubles.

BLACKBERRY

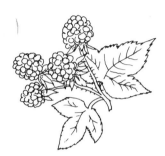

The fruit is rich in mineral salts and is therefore used for anaemia; it is also an astringent, tonic and restorative for the mucous membranes. Blackberry syrup – hot water, honey and blackberries – is good for sore throats, hoarseness and trouble with the upper respiratory tract. Tincture of blackberry is recommended as a gastric tonic: 1 cup of blackberries, covered with 2 pints (1 l.) of alcohol; leave to macerate in the sun or in a warm place for 3 weeks, stirring occasionally; filter and add honey if necessary; take one sherry glass each day.

CABBAGE

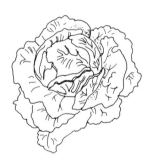

One of the most versatile vegetables – and, surprisingly, most of its effectiveness is through external applications. Chopped cabbage leaves, preferably the greenest, placed between pieces of hot muslin can be used as a compress to relieve liver attacks, intestinal pains, migraines, sprains, rheumatic pains, lumbago, neuralgia, varicose ulcers, eczema, burns and wounds. Poultices should be applied morning and evening to the afflicted area. In the case of a burn or insect bite, a crushed cabbage leaf will reduce the pain and facilitate healing. It will help to heal cuts, sores, pimples, skin outbreaks such as boils and abcesses, superficial infections and swellings. To heal blisters, cook the leaves in milk and apply when cool. As a juice, it is valuable for cirrhosis of the liver, especially when caused by alcoholism, and as a preventive against arthritis and gout. It has also been shown to be successful with gastric ulcers, easing pain quickly and speeding up the healing process; here small regular doses are recommended (up to a total of 18 fluid oz. – 5 dl. – a day) as excessive intake can cause complications. For bronchial infections, coughing and hoarseness, take 1–2 wineglasses of cabbage juice a day with the addition of honey; or as much of the following concentrate as liked: boil six large leaves in 5 cups of water for 30 minutes, sweeten with honey. For a soothing nightcap, try cabbage leaves with a few leaves of sage brewed as a tea; this is also a good gargle for a sore throat.

CARROT

It is now generally acknowledged that carrots increase the number of red blood corpuscles and consequently are one of the best aids for the liver. At Vichy, where they specialize in disorders of the liver, carrots in one form or another are part of every menu. Pure carrot soup is regarded as a worthwhile treatment for a stomach ulcer, and can help constipation too – 2 lb. (1 kg.) carrots to $3\frac{3}{4}$ cups of water, boiled until soft, then liquidized. The high vitamin A content is responsible for many of the good results. It is no myth that it helps eye-strain, not only aiding night-sight but also acting as a restorer for eyes strained by bright lights (vitamin A is destroyed by harsh lighting). As a basic health measure, some advise 1 glass of fresh carrot juice daily, preferably first thing every morning. It protects against colds, flu and bronchitis. Poultices of freshly grated carrots help relieve pain from burns and prevent the formation of blisters. It is important not to scrape carrots for the skin contains a large percentage of the active ingredients; wash and brush only. A cautionary note on carrot juice: don't go overboard and drink more than two glasses a day in the belief that the more the better; some bodies react to excess, and cases of carotene poisoning have been reported.

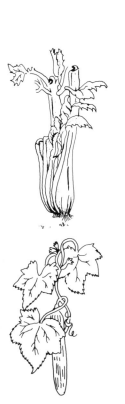

CELERY

Celery is a good source of chlorides, potassium and sodium, but it is the essential oils that put celery on the therapeutic level and have a specific effect on the nervous system. Celery has strong diuretic powers, which means it is useful during any slimming régime, and helps control arthritis, gout and rheumatism. A wineglass of celery juice sweetened with a tablespoon of honey will reduce the appetite when taken before meals. Eaten raw at the end of a meal, it acts as a digestive, and has the reputation of being a natural antacid. As a poultice – grated raw and combined with linseed – it helps swollen glands.

CUCUMBER

Gets rid of excess fluid and any toxic matter in the body. It is therefore of prime interest to dieters (a minimum of 3 wineglasses of juice a day). Combined with carrot and celery juice, it is good for all rheumatic conditions. It is, however, mainly used as an external application to aid the skin (see Beauty Preparations, pages 156ff).

FIG

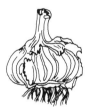

Mainly used dried, the fig helps constipation, relieves chest complaints and is a remedy for colds and throat conditions. Its use as a laxative is well known: the seeds stimulate the bowels into action. Soak 6 dried figs in tepid water, leave overnight and eat first thing in the morning; also drink the water. A decoction of figs can be taken for pulmonary infections, used as a gargle for throat irritations and as a mouthwash for gum disorders such as abscesses or gingivitis. Boil 6 figs in 2 pints (1 l.) water or milk for five minutes, strain. Externally, a poultice of fresh figs or dried figs cooked in milk can soothe burns and draw abscesses and boils to a head. To help chilblains and haemorrhoids, roast figs in the oven, pulverize and mix with honey; use lightly.

GARLIC

This plant has become synonymous with health, energy and longevity. It has two outstanding medical properties: it helps open up blood vessels, thus aiding many maladies connected with circulation, and it is a strong antibiotic. For centuries it has been a common remedy for colds, coughs, bronchitis and sore throats as it induces perspiration and stimulates energy. One of the best ways to take it is by drinking milk in which you have boiled cloves of garlic. For arthritis, rheumatism, sciatica and sinus infections, mash 2 garlic cloves with a teaspoon of honey and take for three or four nights in succession. Garlic browned in butter and honey helps kidney and bladder troubles. Infused in milk or water, it is recommended for reducing blood pressure and relieving headaches. Animal studies have shown improvement in arteriosclerosis conditions; Italians (who eat garlic with almost everything) have a lower incidence of heart disease than most Europeans. Garlic also brings relief in cases of indigestion, intestinal infections and liver disorders. It has long been recognized as one of the best natural remedies for getting rid of worms because of the high allicin content of the oil.

Here is a good garlic tonic: mince 2 garlic cloves and steep in a glass of white wine for 3 days; take a teaspoon first thing every morning. Or steep chopped garlic in alcohol in the ratio of one part garlic to two of alcohol.

Allow to stand in the warmth (sunlight or near a stove) for 2 weeks; strain. Begin by taking 2 drops in a glass of warm water before lunch or dinner (once a day only) and each successive day increase the dose by one drop until a maximum of 25 is reached; then reverse the procedure, returning drop by drop to 1. This tonic can be taken several times a year, but allow an interval of six weeks between treatments.

An ointment can be made by crushing 2 cloves of garlic and blending it in 2 tablespoons of lard. This can be rubbed or massaged into areas of rheumatic pain or neuritis; it also helps to ease sprains and muscular pains.

Garlic is also an antiseptic; it has a powerful effect on healing wounds and was much in demand during the First World War. It can also be applied to insect stings and bites – mash a clove, or extract the juice, and mix with small amounts of hot water or honey.

HORSE-RADISH

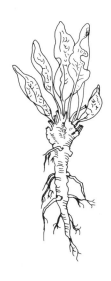

One of the more potent diuretics, with a stimulating effect on the blood capillaries and so useful in the treatment of kidney conditions: chop 1 oz. (30 g.) of fresh horse-radish root, add ½ oz. (15 g.) bruised mustard seed and a pint (6 dl.) of boiling water; cover and steep for 5 hours; strain and take 3 tablespoons a day. Horse-radish can be added to other vegetable juices to stimulate digestion and help urine pass through weak kidneys. It can be also mixed with white wine or made into a sauce by shredding and mashing the root and adding lemon juice. A very good solvent for mucus in the nose and sinus: take half a teaspoon of horse-radish sauce morning and early evening. Do not drink or eat anything for 15 minutes afterwards – there is a feeling of clearance in the head, the eyes may stream and sometimes there is sweating. Small doses only; large amounts could damage the lining of the stomach and intestines. It may take some time to clear the passages, even months for a severe case. A syrup made of grated horse-radish, honey and water can be taken for hoarseness. Externally, a compress made with grated horse-radish mixed with a little water produces heat and relieves rheumatic pains, neuralgia and stiffness.

LEMON

Probably the most valuable of all fruits for preserving health. Because of its high vitamin C content it has been used for hundreds of years as a protection against scurvy. It can neutralize harmful and infectious bacteria, which is why in many hot climates the juice of a lemon is a last-minute addition to meat, fish and vegetable dishes. On raw oysters it destroys 90 per cent of the bacteria within 15 minutes. Lemon juice is used in all kinds of infections of the respiratory tract and as a general tonic – the juice should be diluted with water, sweetened with honey if desired; there is no need to worry about drinking too much in this form. It is valuable as a cooling drink in fevers and when temperatures are high it is advisable to take regular drinks to prevent dehydration. It is a cure for stubborn hiccoughs and helpful in jaundice – recent research indicates that lemon juice may aid in the regeneration of the liver, balancing the harmful effects of alcohol. Those who wish to lose weight or to avoid putting on weight should drink it first thing in the morning diluted with hot or cold water or mineral water. It is a good astringent and may be used as a gargle for a sore throat, in uterine haemorrhage after delivery or as a sunburn lotion.

LETTUCE

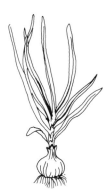

Its rich mineral content, including iodine, phosphorus, iron, copper, cobalt, zinc, calcium, manganese and potassium, make it one of the best restorers of the body's mineral balance. The outer green leaves are the most beneficial. It is good for the nervous system as it has calming effect. It is also prescribed for gastric spasms and palpitations and can be used as a sedative; a small lettuce, simmered in 1 pint (6 dl.) of water for 15 minutes, makes a helpful night drink for insomniacs.

ONION

The oils that give the onion its pungency are therapeutic agents which have an excellent internal and external germicidal effect. The onion has much the same powers as garlic, but to a lesser degree; little of its value is lost in cooking. It has a normalizing influence on the nervous system and stimulates the growth of beneficial bacteria in the intestines. It aids digestion and secretion of bile; it also can lower blood pressure. It is a standard remedy against colds and catarrh, as well as being a good general tonic: to 5 oz. (150 g.) grated onion mixed with $3\frac{1}{2}$ oz. (100 g.) honey, add 2 pints (1 l.) white wine; cover and steep for 2 weeks, strain; take 4 teaspoons a day. A raw onion is recommended for rheumatism. Externally the raw juice can relieve painful joints; poultices of raw mashed onion help draw out foreign matter from infected areas; a slice of fresh onion rubbed on the infected area daily can clear up an abscess, because the onion has the power to absorb poisons. (Never eat or cook decayed onions – they are contaminated.)

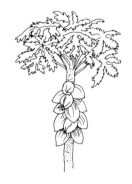

PAPAYA

Also known as paw-paw. This is extremely rich in the enzymes that make the digestion of protein possible. An infusion of the fruit and leaves will make the toughest meat tender, a fact that illustrates its digestive value. Combined with cucumber juice it is an efficient general cleanser: during a 12-hour period, take, once every hour, $\frac{1}{4}$ pint (1·5 dl.) papaya juice and $\frac{1}{4}$ pint (1·5 dl.) cucumber juice alternately. Eaten regularly, the papaya can be helpful in the prevention of kidney stones. Mixed with a boiled egg yolk it can help cirrhosis of the liver. With honey it is good for urinary disorders and is a tonic for the heart, liver and blood. The skin is used as a special external treatment for wounds and infections that fail to heal properly or quickly. It has been claimed that papaya has rejuvenating properties, especially with regard to stalling premature ageing – this may be due to its ability to keep the digestive system in peak condition.

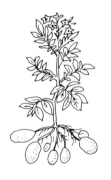

POTATO

The important nutrients lie just under the skin so the healthy way to eat potatoes is scrubbed and baked or boiled, not peeled. In winter, it is one of the most useful sources of vitamin C; it also contains valuable B vitamins and a rich supply of potassium. The juice is an antacid and soothing to the gastric tract so it is used to treat duodenal and gastric ulcers as well as gastritis. Recently it has successfully been used to treat rheumatism and gout. The juice can be combined with carrot juice for a more pleasant taste – $\frac{1}{2}$ wineglass three or four times a day for at least a month. Grated raw potato relieves the pains of burn and sunburn. Slices of raw potato on the forehead soothe headaches; they can relieve bags under the eyes and puffy lids.

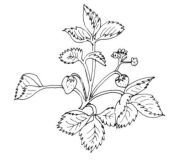

STRAWBERRY

Because of its very high iron content it is used in the treatment of anaemia. It also helps to lower blood pressure. The rich supply of salicylic acid aids the functions of the liver, kidneys and joints, and it is a good detoxifying agent.

Large quantities of strawberries (a diet of almost nothing else) have been known to cure gout. Chronic gastroenteritis can be helped by eating 10-18 oz. (300-500 g.) of strawberries a day for a month. The seeds aid constipation as they are not broken down by gastric juices and act as an irritant to stimulate bowel movements.

WATERCRESS

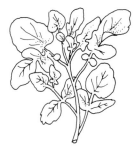

Rich in sulphur, nitrogen and iodine, watercress is one of the finest blood purifiers, and is also an excellent source of vitamins A and C. It is good as a general tonic for liver and kidney troubles. It makes a particularly effective spring tonic: dilute the juice in water (1 part juice to 5 parts water) and take 2 teaspoons eight times a day for a minimum of 2 weeks. Watercress is useful in skin diseases – apply the juice to troubled areas at night and wash away in the morning.

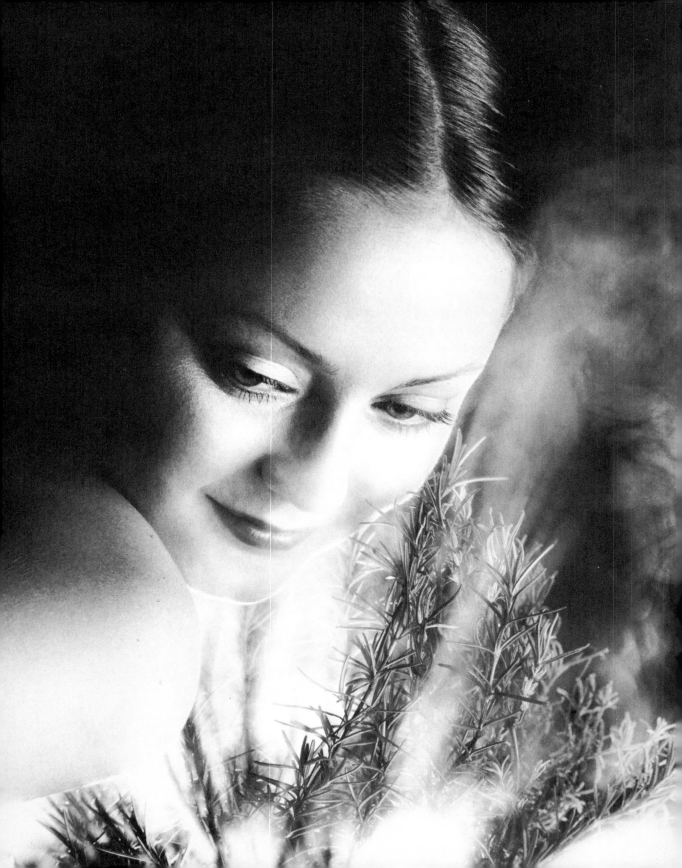

2

HERBS AND TISANES

A group of easily obtainable herbs has traditionally formed the core of domestic health aids, helping common ailments such as colds, chills, influenza, stomach and digestion troubles, bronchitis and rheumatic conditions. They are recommended as preventive measures and a valid alternative to drugs; it is possible to treat common maladies at home with herbs in their gentlest form as infusions, decoctions, tonics, wines and syrups or as a mild tisane. Herbal tinctures and extracts are too potent for the amateur, requiring consultation and prescription by a qualified herbalist or homoeopathic practitioner.

For sensible prevention and limited doctoring, you need look no further than the nineteen herbs listed below. Their power is expelled through liquid and heat or both. These are called infusions, decoctions and macerations, while a tisane (or herb tea) is simply a drink containing a lower proportion of the medicinal herbal substance. The same group of herbs is also featured in the section on cookery (pages 240–41), which gives ideas for using them in the preparation of food. Their medicinal value is then at its lowest, but they nevertheless counteract any adverse aspects (such as heaviness or fatty content) and they are the natural, healthy way of adding flavour.

GATHERING

Plants should be picked at the time of full maturity, preferably on a dry and sunny day in the morning – though not too early because of the possibility of dew. Damp plants rapidly deteriorate and become almost valueless. It is important to think about the time of maturity for the part you need. For example, the roots are usually at their most beneficial in the spring before the shoots use up the stored goodness; the leaves and flowers are at their zenith in the summer; the berries in the autumn; bark should be taken from a young tree. Herbs purchased commercially should be in a tightly sealed container. (Tea-bag herbs for tisanes may have lost some of their potency.)

DRYING

This is very important, because herbs will be adversely affected if they are not dried correctly. Leaves, flowers and berries should be dried in a ventilated area, in the shade, not the sun. (Heat and brightness can destroy essential oils.) They should be separated and spread out immediately after gathering; never wash or clean in any way beforehand. Each day turn them over so that drying is even. When thoroughly dried, they can be cut or broken up for storing. Roots are dried in a different way; they must be washed as soon as they are collected and can be put into the sun for a few hours on the first day and afterwards kept in the shade. It is better to cut or slice the root before further drying, as it is almost impossible to do so later.

STORING

Make sure the herbs are thoroughly dry, as any trace of dampness will spread and ruin all. They should be stored away from the air and in a dry dark place. The best containers are glass jars, with cork stoppers, as they enable you to check on the contents. Avoid plastic wrappings.

PREPARATION

There are three ways to prepare herbs at home: infusion, decoction and maceration. The infusion and tisane (a weak infusion) should be made with the purest possible water, a mild mineral water is best if local water is contaminated: a heavy limestone content in water prevents herbs from releasing their active ingredients. An infusion or decoction should not be prepared too long in advance; after twenty-four hours the power diminishes. They should not be reheated.

Infusion

An infusion is prepared by pouring boiling water over bruised roots, bark, leaves, flowers or seeds in the proportion of 1 pint (6 dl.) of water to 1 oz. (30 g.) of the herb. Use glass, china or earthenware containers. Cover and allow to steep for a minimum of 15 minutes. Strain the infusion before use. (These quantities are average and can be taken as a general rule unless otherwise specified.)

Tisane

A mild infusion, averaging ½ oz. (15 g.) of the herb to 1 pint (6 dl.) water. Allow to steep for 5 to 15 minutes.

Decoction

Some herbs, particularly when the root and bark are the parts used, only expel the valuable matter when boiled. Cold water is added to the given amount of the herb, and they are then boiled together for about 30 minutes, cooled and strained. Sometimes extra water needs to be added during the boiling. Use glass, enamel or earthenware pans.

Maceration

The herb is soaked in oil, wine, vinegar or alcohol for a specified length of time, which could be anything from a few hours to several weeks. These usually serve as tonics and are taken in small doses.

Ointments and Poultices

Herbs for these are prepared as an infusion or decoction but in greater strength. For a poultice, gauze pads are soaked in the herbal liquid, or the herb itself is sandwiched between hot damp pieces of gauze – it is the liquid and vapour that heal. To make an ointment, take 1 part of the liquid to 4 parts of a fat such as lard, anhydrous lanolin or Vaseline and mix well together.

DOSAGE

In the following guide, definite amounts are usually given, but in general a wineglass of an infusion or decoction can be taken three times a day (every 4 hours during waking hours). A tisane can be drunk as often as liked, as a substitute for a cup of tea or coffee. A sherry glass of a wine or tonic syrup (made by maceration) may also be taken three times a day, before or during meals. To drink more is not necessarily better; herbs are slow correctors and excess quantities are not desirable.

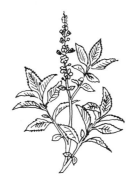

AGRIMONY

This herb has a slightly bitter taste, and is used internally as an infusion or as a component in herbal tea mixtures. It acts as an astringent, tonic and diuretic, regulating the stomach and liver functions, including the gall bladder. It is considered a good safe stomach tonic, helping assimilation of food. The leaves are used to make a tisane, taken once a day for maintenance and three or four times a day as a treatment. It has a reputation for helping to cure jaundice and other liver complaints: infuse 6 oz. of the crown of the root in a quart of boiling water (150 g. root to 1 l. water), allow to steep for 15 minutes, sweeten with honey; drink ½ pint (3 dl.) three times a day. It is also used as a gargle for inflammation of the throat and tonsillitis: boil 4 oz. dried leaves in a quart of water (100 g. leaves to 1 l. water) until liquid is reduced by a third; gargle five times a day; if too bitter add a little honey.

Externally it can help to heal wounds, varicose ulcers and sprains: boil 8 oz. of dried leaves in a quart of water (200 g. leaves to 1 l. water) for 5 minutes; leave to infuse for an hour, clean the wounds with the liquid and then apply compresses. The same decoction can be used to clear skin rashes and break-outs.

It flowers from June to August and for medicinal purposes should be gathered before the seeds appear.

ANGELICA

A remedy for colds, coughs, pleurisy, wind and diseases of the urinary organs. It can also stimulate the secretion of gastric juices. Small doses are imperative as excess adversely affects the central nervous system. It should never be taken by anyone with diabetes as it causes an increase of sugar. It is usually taken as an infusion: 1 oz. (30 g.) angelica root, finely chopped, covered with a pint (6 dl.) of boiling water; steep for 30 minutes and drink 2 tablespoons three or four times a day. It can be used alone or in herbal tea mixtures to stimulate the appetite, act as a tonic and help anaemia. It is said to be effective in cases of nervous asthma or smokers' cough. A drink widely recommended in Europe for typhus fever (and for other feverish conditions too) is 6 oz. angelica root, thinly sliced, infused in a quart of boiling water for 30 minutes, strain, add juice of 2 lemons, 4 oz. honey and $\frac{1}{2}$ gill brandy (150 g. angelica root, 1 l. water, juice of 2 lemons, 100 g. honey and 4 tablespoons brandy). Take 2 tablespoons morning and night and three or four times during the day.

Externally it can help badly healing wounds, varicose ulcers and sprains: boil 8 oz. dried leaves in a quart of water (200 g. leaves to 1 l. water) for 5 minutes, leave to infuse for an hour. Clean wounds with this liquid, then apply compresses. The same liquid can be used to clear skin rashes. Fresh leaves, crushed and applied as a poultice are helpful for lung and chest diseases. The roots and leaves are employed medically, and sometimes the seeds as well.

The roots should be dug up in the autumn of the first year of growth. When thick, slice longitudinally to quicken the drying process. The whole herb should be gathered in June, and the leaves stripped for drying (the stem is mostly used in confectionery). The seeds should be collected when ripe and dried.

BASIL

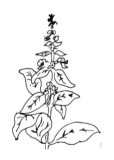

Basil, aromatic and carminative, serves as a non-toxic kind of tranquillizer and is prescribed for mild nervous disorders. Dried leaves in the form of snuff can cure nervous headaches. It is good for all obstructions of the internal organs; it helps stomach disorders, particularly those of nervous origin, arrests vomiting and allays nausea. As a tea it should be drunk two or three times a day after meals: 8 oz. leaves or flowering tips covered with a quart of boiling water (200 g. leaves to 1 l. boiling water), infuse for 10 minutes. As a tonic wine for digestion: macerate a handful of leaves in a quart (1 l.) of wine for 3 days, strain; take a small wineglass after each meal. This wine can be combined with an equal amount of olive oil to relieve persistent constipation – 1 tablespoon of each mixed together, three or four times a day. A tisane of basil sweetened with a generous amount of honey aids and speeds up the elimination of mucous in catarrh of the chest and obstruction of mucous in the lungs. The juice of fresh leaves helps inflammations of the ear – use just a few drops. The juice can also be put on wasp stings.

BAY

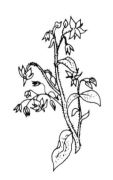

The leaves of the bay tree are very aromatic and strong. The leaves, berries and oil have excitant and narcotic properties, and can stimulate the appetite and relieve pain. Use the leaves (gathered fresh year-round or dried) as an infusion: 1 or 2 leaves left in hot tea for 10 minutes; or in wine – leave for 1 hour in a warm place. When using dried leaves to make a tea, steep 2 oz. crushed leaves in a quart of boiling water (50 g. leaves to 1 l. water) for 10 minutes. A cup of this tea can also be drunk immediately after meals to aid digestion. A bay leaf chewed before meals encourages the secretion of saliva and so helps digestion. Dried and powdered leaves act as a preventive against intermittent fevers: leave 15 grains (1 g.) powder to macerate in a wineglass of cold water for 10 hours; drink 2 hours prior to the expected bout of fever. For rheumatism and fever take a decoction of the berries: boil 1 oz. (30 g.) pitted crushed berries for 5 minutes in 1¾ pints (1 l.) water and allow to infuse for 10 minutes; take 3 cups a day, before or between meals. Oil of bay contains a high percentage of oxygenated compounds and is applied externally for sprains and bruises; it is sometimes used as ear drops.

BORAGE

Contains potassium and calcium combined with mineral acids. The fresh leaves provide 30 per cent nitrate of potash, the dried only 3 per cent. The stems and leaves yield a great deal of saline mucilage. It is these salts that account for the healing properties of borage, making it a blood purifier, nerve tonic and treatment for palpitations of the heart and hysteria. Recent knowledge shows that borage tends to activate the adrenal gland. It is traditionally reputed to relieve depression and instigate feelings of optimism. A quick tisane can be brewed from a teaspoon of dried borage leaves (or 1 tablespoon chopped fresh leaves) and a cup of boiling water; infuse for a few minutes, sweeten with honey. For fevers due to chills, influenza and contagious diseases such as measles, chicken-pox and scarlet fever, a wineglass of the infusion should be sipped three or four times a day: 2 oz. (60 g.) leaves to $1\frac{3}{4}$ pints (1 l.) boiling water, infused for half an hour. Compresses made from the leaves help relieve congestion of the veins, particularly in the legs.

The flowers yield an excellent honey, and are also used medicinally, though to a smaller extent than the leaves. Gather the plant when it is coming into flower (May or June); strip the leaves and flowers from the stem and dry both. Pick on a fine day when the sun has dried the dew.

BURDOCK

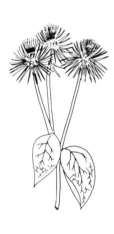

The leaves, root and seeds are all used for medicinal purposes. It is one of the superior blood purifiers and an aid for skin diseases – it has often cured eczema. An infusion of the leaves – a tablespoon to a cup of boiling water – gives strength and tone to the stomach. The tisane is cleansing and is often used to relieve stones in the kidneys or bladder. A mixture of dandelion and burdock tea is a blood purifier and tonic. The anti-scorbutic properties of the root make it effective for boils, scurvy and rheumatic conditions. To make a decoction of the root use 1 oz. (30 g.) to $1\frac{1}{2}$ pints (9 dl.) water, boil down to a pint (6 dl.) and take 3–4 wineglasses in the course of the day. Also recommended for diabetes as it can lower the blood sugar level. For rheumatic conditions slice 2 oz. (60 g.) fresh root, cover with 5 pints (3 l.) of boiling water; leave until cold, strain, add $\frac{7}{8}$ pint (5 dl.) milk and sweeten with 5 tablespoons honey. Drink a third on rising, a third at midday and the remaining third in the evening. If the joints are particularly sore, apply poultices of the fresh leaves.

The seeds are so oily that they affect both the sebaceous and sudoriferous glands. A medicinal fluid extract is used to treat skin diseases. An infusion or decoction of the seeds is used for dropsy, particularly in cases where the nervous system is off-balance; it is good for all kidney troubles – take before meals.

Externally a poultice of the mashed leaves boiled for 5 minutes in lightly salted water is a resolvent for tumours and swellings caused by gout; it will also relieve bruises and inflamed surfaces. A decoction of the seeds can be applied as a healing wash for ulcers and scaly skin disorders. It is claimed that it is helpful in the growth of hair: repeatedly rub into the scalp a lotion made from 1 oz. fresh leaves boiled in $2\frac{1}{2}$ cups water (30 g. leaves to 1 l. water) for 5 minutes; allow to steep and cool before use; or use a 1:1 mixture of the above lotion and wine vinegar, and rub into the scalp morning and evening.

CAMOMILE

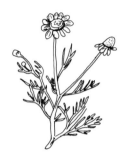

One of the oldest herbs and a special favourite amongst herbalists. The entire plant is odoriferous but the medicinal value lies mostly in the flower heads, where the volatile oil is an important element. It is used internally in the form of an infusion: 1 oz. (30 g.) flowers to 1 pint (6 dl.) boiling water. Allow to steep for 10 minutes, but cover the container to prevent the escape of the active volatile ingredients. It can be taken regularly in doses from a tablespoon to a cup. It is excellent for all nervous conditions as it has the capacity to calm, inducing sleep and preventing nightmares. This tisane also relieves indigestion, pains in the stomach and in particular menstrual cramps. It is said to help kidney, spleen and bladder troubles.

Externally it can be applied as a compress to swellings and congested neuralgia; of special note is the capacity of a poultice to reduce facial swellings due to abscesses – steep the gauze-wrapped flowers in boiling water before applying. To help inflammation of the eyelids, conjunctivitis and skin infections, bathe with the following decoction (or apply in compresses): 2 oz. (60 g.) flowers to $1\frac{3}{4}$ pints (1 l.) water, bring to the boil and leave covered to infuse for 20 minutes. This lotion may be added to the bath to relax and counteract tiredness; it will also relieve haemorrhoids and rheumatic pains.

COMFREY

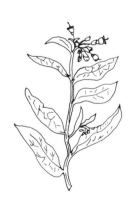

For hundreds of years comfrey has been considered one of the most valuable natural healing plants. The most important element in comfrey is allantoin, which appears to stimulate all growth and multiplication of cells, thus strengthening skin tissues and helping to heal lesions, particularly ulcers. In 1936 an English physician, Charles J. Macalister, compiled a treatise on comfrey and its success in healing skin ulcers. Chemical research revealed that the active part was allantoin. This is also found in the urine of pregnant women and in plant life in the areas connected with growth and development; it is a component of mother's milk. Dr Macalister came to the conclusion that allantoin provided the means for development of cells, which in terms of healing also meant repair. When young the horizontal roots of the plant contain a high percentage of allantoin, which gradually decreases so that by summer, when mature, there is practically none in the root but a lot in the buds, leaves and shoots. This confirms that the plant draws on the allantoin for cell proliferation. An infusion is made from 1 oz. (30 g.) comfrey covered by 1 pint (6 dl.) boiling water and steeped for 15 minutes. It is best to use fresh leaves, though a tisane can be made from 1 teaspoon dried leaves in a cup of hot water. A decoction of the root is made by crushing and simmering 1 oz. (30 g.) in 1 quart (1 l.) of water for 30 minutes. This has long been given for intestinal troubles, and is a mild, effective remedy for diarrhoea, dysentery and stomach ulcers. It is a traditional aid for lung troubles and whooping cough, the root being more efficient than the leaves. It is a traditional remedy for everything from consumption to haemorrhoids. A hot strong brew is drunk to help bad bruises, swellings, sprains and boils.

Externally the young leaves are used as prime healers. A compress is the general method: chop up leaves and infuse with boiling water; when cool place between two layers of gauze. The leaves have the ability to reduce swelling, so facilitating the union of the bones in the case of fractures. In addition, poultices are used for wounds, ulcers, burns and gangrene. If repeated applications are necessary, it is advisable to first smear the skin with lanolin to avoid irritation. Comfrey mixed with vitamin E or wheatgerm provides a quick-action ointment for healing.

ELDER

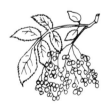

The elder has been well-known in domestic medicine since the days of Hippocrates. All parts of the tree are used – bark, leaves, flowers and berries. An infusion of the bark acts as a strong purgative: 1 oz. (30 g.) steeped in 1 pint (6 dl.) boiling water for 15 minutes, to be taken in wineglass doses. Ideally the bark should be collected from young trees in the autumn; it should be dried in the sun, and is ready for use when light grey and corky on the outside, white and smooth underneath. The leaves can be used fresh or dry – picked in June and July, early in the morning and in fine weather.

The leaves are laxative, purgative and diuretic; make an infusion with a tablespoon of chopped leaves in a cup of boiling water and allow to steep for a minimum of 30 minutes; alternatively, boil fresh leaves in milk, in the same proportions. A strong, cooled infusion helps inflammation of the eyes.

A cool infusion of the leaves when dabbed on the skin helps keep away mosquitoes and other insects. The leaves when boiled with linseed oil until soft can be applied externally to heal piles. A remedy for bruises, sprains and chilblains is green elder ointment: $1\frac{1}{2}$ oz. (45 g.) fresh elder leaves, 2 oz. (60 g.) lard or anhydrous lanolin, $\frac{1}{2}$ oz. (15 g.) grated suet; melt lard and suet, add chopped leaves and simmer until the leaves have lost their colour; strain. An ointment combining other herbs is claimed to be particularly effective for swellings, tumours and wounds: chop into small pieces 2 oz. (60 g.) elder leaves, 1 oz. (30 g.) plantain leaves, $\frac{1}{2}$ oz. (15 g.) ground ivy, 1 oz. (30 g.) wormwood and add to 1 lb. (500 g.) of melted lard or anhydrous lanolin; simmer over a low flame until the herbs are crisp; strain.

The flowers of elder can be used fresh or dried though the flowering season only lasts three weeks in June. An infusion helps bronchial and pulmonary afflictions, scarlet fever, measles and other eruptive diseases. It is a tried and true remedy for colds and throat troubles as it induces perspiration: an infusion should be taken on going to bed. One of the best cures for influenza in its first stage is a strong infusion of dried elder blossoms and peppermint: put $\frac{1}{2}$ cup of each in a container, infuse with $1\frac{1}{2}$ pints (9 dl.) boiling water and steep for 30 minutes. A tisane of the flowers is a spring tonic and blood purifier: to be taken every morning before breakfast. Elder flowers make a good vinegar gargle for sore throats: put $\frac{1}{2}$ lb. (250 g.) dried flowers in a closed glass container with $\frac{1}{2}$ pint (3 dl.) of cider vinegar; keep in a warm place for 8 days, shaking from time to time. Externally, a strong infusion of flowers (brewed for 1 hour) can be applied as a compress to tumours, boils and skin break-outs. The same infusion mixed with warm lard is a dressing for wounds, burns and scalds.

The berries can be made into a wine or syrup to help colds, bronchitis, influenza and asthma. For the wine recipe see page 289; for the syrup, stew the ripe berries in a little water for 15 minutes, strain; to each 2 quarts (2·3 l.) add 8 whole cloves and $\frac{1}{4}$ oz. (7 g.) ginger; boil for 1 hour, strain before bottling. The wine or the syrup can be taken before all meals – one wineglass, with hot water if desired.

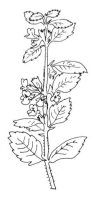

LEMON BALM

The leaves and flowering tops are used, but if dried should be kept in a sealed container, though not for more than a year. A tisane is made from 1 oz. (30 g.) of the herb covered with 1 pint (6 dl.) boiling water, infused for 15 minutes. This can be taken frequently (when cool) for fever, influenza and catarrh. It is a soothing and relaxing drink and is therefore used to help disorders stemming from a nervous condition – agitation, headaches, palpitation, irritability, insomnia. It soothes tension, helps depression and eases digestive troubles stemming from nerves. It is specially helpful for menstrual cramps and uterine pains – up to 6 cups of the tea a day; 10 to 15 drops of balm on a lump of sugar will stem fainting, nausea and vomiting. Externally it is an effective dressing for wounds; it is now scientifically recognized that the balsamic oils of aromatic plants make excellent surgical dressings.

MALLOW

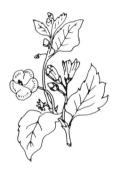

The European marsh mallow belongs to a large and important plant family, particularly prevalent in tropical regions. The root, leaves and flowers are all of medicinal value because of the high content of mucilage. It is used for inflammation and irritation of the alimentary canal and the urinary and respiratory organs; also for colds, coughs, bronchitis, gastritis, cystitis and constipation. An infusion is made by pouring 2 pints of boiling water over 2 oz. of leaves and flowers (1 l. water to 50 g. leaves), allowing it to stand covered for an hour; take 4 cups daily. A decoction of the root is particularly effective in painful complaints of the urinary system: 5 pints (3 l.) water to 4 oz. (120 g.) dried root, chopped finely, boil until liquid is reduced to 3 pints (1·7 l.), strain; take 3 or 4 wineglasses a day. This decoction also helps cure bruises, sprains and muscle aches. Boiled in wine or milk, the powdered root will relieve chest colds and coughs. Another decoction of the root – 2 oz. to 2 pints of water (50 g. to 1 l. water) – is used as a gargle for sore throats and tonsillitis and as a mouthwash for abscesses and gingivitis. It is also recommended as a very hot inhalation for sinusitis.

Externally a poultice of the leaves or the fresh chopped root aids burns, boils, carbuncles and reduces inflammation and swelling.

MARJORAM

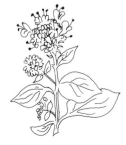

The active parts are found in the leaves, which are at their peak just before the flowering period, any time from July to September. An infusion is made from 1 teaspoon marjoram leaves covered with 1 cup boiling water. It is taken for digestive upsets, colic, flatulence and diarrhoea and can also stimulate the secretion of bile. It is good as a tonic and is recommended for loss of appetite. It should not be drunk during pregnancy. However, a tisane can help normalize irregular menstruation; take 4 cups a day three or four days before the calculated date of the period. A tea of wild marjoram (oregano) prevents sea-sickness and acts as a sedative. Compresses of the infusion are used to relieve the pain of swollen rheumatic joints but the oil extract usually has a greater effect. The oil is used as an external application for sprains and bruises and a drop or two on the tooth and gum can also alleviate toothache. In powdered form it is a component of snuff and can also be taken on its own.

MINT

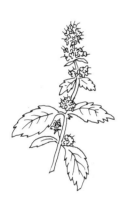

There are three chief varieties of mint – spearmint (the garden genre), peppermint and pennyroyal, but they have much in common and have been held in medical esteem for centuries. Spearmint is mostly used for culinary purposes and is less potent than peppermint. It is therefore better suited for children: an infusion made by pouring 1 pint (6 dl.) boiling water on 1 oz. (30 g.) of the dried herb should be taken in sherry-glass doses. It helps allay nausea and vomiting and will relieve the pain of colic.

The oil from peppermint is considered one of the most important of the volatile oils. Its chief constituent is menthol, which has a penetrating odour and cooling taste and provides the medicinal value. It is soothing as well as stimulating to the whole of the digestive system. The oil extract is the most powerful, but the leaves (gathered from June to August) release appreciable amounts of menthol in infusions and decoctions. These can be taken in a variety of strengths, sipped hot and slowly; the average proportions are: 1 oz. (30 g.) dried leaves to 1 pint (6 dl.) boiling water, or 6 fresh leaves to 1 cup boiling water. It can relieve pains in the alimentary canal due to digestive disturbances, is a quick antidote for sudden pains and cramp in the abdomen and in fact helps any intestinal and gastric complaint, flatulence, gall bladder disorders and spasms. Wide use is made of peppermint for cholera and severe diarrhoea.

Mint can also tone up the nervous system and is therefore prescribed for general listlessness, heart palpitations and to counteract the enervation of hot weather. It is one of the best remedies for headaches and can also be used freely as a tea to ward off colds and influenza; an infusion of equal parts peppermint and elder flowers will swiftly get rid of a cold.

Externally, inhalations – 2 oz. leaves to a quart of boiling water (50 g. leaves to 1 l. water) – are effective for respiratory troubles such as bronchitis, coughs and asthma; better results are obtained if inhalation and regular drinks of a strong infusion are used in conjunction. Fresh or dried leaves, softened in warm water and applied as compresses help rheumatic, joint and muscular pains and gout. This also minimizes headache and migraine pains – even fresh bruised leaves placed directly on the forehead can be effective.

PARSLEY

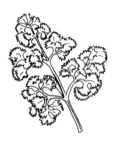

Although one of the most common herbs, parsley is therapeutically underrated. It is rich in iron, calcium, vitamins and trace elements – it actually contains more vitamin C than any other common culinary vegetable, and provides as much vitamin A as carrots. All parts of the plant are used – root, leaves and seeds, preferably fresh. The medicinal value is due to the presence of apiol, which is particularly helpful for disorders of the menstrual cycle, whether painful or absent, and urinary upsets and infections, including stones and decreased flow of urine: boil 4 oz. seed, root or leaves in a quart of water (100 g. in 1 l. water) for 5 minutes, steep for 20 minutes. Take 1 wineglass before all meals. The same decoction is recommended as a diuretic for gout and rheumatism, and because of its high mineral and vitamin content, it can be drunk regularly as a tonic to alleviate anaemia. The dried root in decoction – 2 oz. boiled in a quart of water (50 g. in 1 l. water) for 3 minutes, steeped for 10 minutes – particularly stimulates kidney function and is therefore prescribed for all ailments where retention of water and toxic matter is the problem; take a cupful before each meal. For loss of appetite, a tea of parsley leaves can be substituted for other beverages. Parsley juice combined with warm milk can help asthma, bronchitis and laryngitis.

Externally the crushed fresh leaves will relieve stings and insect bites; eye irritations may respond to compresses of bruised leaves or 1 drop of fresh juice applied three times a day. Cooked in wine, the leaves can be used as a warm poultice on bruises and sprains. Equal parts of parsley juice and 140° proof alcohol can help neuralgia – apply with finger and rub in. An infusion of 4 oz. parsley seeds to a quart of water (100 g. parsley seeds to 1 l. water) is a beneficial douche for vaginal infections.

ROSEMARY

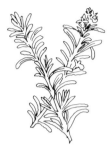

The leaves and flowering tops are used; both yield their medicinal qualities in part only in water and entirely in wine or vinegar. Rosemary is a strong stimulant, quickening the senses and acting as a catalyst on the brain and nervous system, and is therefore a good remedy for headaches caused by weak circulation. It also relieves nervous depression and helps stomach upsets and malfunction of the liver and gall bladder. Rosemary tea should be taken warm, a cup after each meal except in the case of liver complaints, when it should be drunk before eating: 2 oz. to a quart of boiling water (50 g. to 1 l. water). A rosemary wine given in small quantities – a sherry glass twice a day with main meals – acts positively in cases of a weak heart and palpitation and can also relieve water retention by stimulating the kidneys: chop up 4 oz. fresh sprigs of rosemary and macerate in a quart of white wine (100 g. rosemary to 1 l. wine) for a minimum of 5 days; a light Bordeaux or Chianti red wine can be used if preferred. Rosemary wine is a good tonic for the entire system.

Externally rosemary is used as a poultice to treat rheumatic pains or bruises; as a lotion it acts as a skin or hair tonic (see Beauty Preparations pages 168, 205ff) and can help get rid of puffiness under the eyes. Wide use is made of rosemary oil in ointments and liniments to alleviate pain in rheumatism of the muscles and joints. An infusion of leaves is a good mouthwash for gums, bad breath or a sore throat.

SAGE

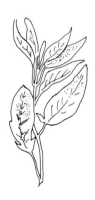

Sage has the reputation of being a stimulant for the nervous system and brain but it is primarily a digestive, aiding any weakness of the stomach, especially if of a nervous origin. It activates circulation and sustains the heart so is of service to convalescents and those afflicted with overstrain and general breakdowns. It also has a regulating effect on the hormones and is important for pregnant women and during the menopause. The Chinese had great faith in the overall benefits of drinking sage tea daily, while the Italians have always considered it a general preventive medicine. An infusion is made from 3 dried or fresh leaves to a cup of boiling water, steeped for 5 minutes; 2 or 3 cups a day are recommended. It can be taken as a wine after meals: macerate 4 oz. sage (fresh or dried) in a quart of white wine (100 g. sage to 1 l. wine) for a week; take a sherry glass after meals.

Externally a decoction of sage can be used as a gargle for sore and ulcerated throats, as well as a mouthwash for dental inflammations and abscesses: use $\frac{3}{4}$ oz. to a quart of water (20 g. to 1 l. water), boil for 5 minutes and steep for 10 minutes. This same decoction makes a good vaginal douche. An alternative for gargling and mouth problems is: 1 sherry glass port, 1 tablespoon cider vinegar, 6 sage leaves and 2 teaspoons honey simmered for 5 minutes. A strong decoction – 4 oz. to a quart of water (100 g. to 1 l. water), boiled for 5 minutes – can be applied as a compress to eczema, spots and badly healing sores. To help sprains: use $\frac{1}{2}$ cup crushed sage leaves boiled in a cup of water for 5 minutes. A sage ointment can be massaged twice daily into stiff joints and muscles, rheumatic and gout areas: pulverize 3 cups fresh leaves (in a mortar) and mix with 1 lb. (500 g.) lard or anhydrous lanolin; boil over a low heat until the leaves appear dehydrated and strain through a fine cloth.

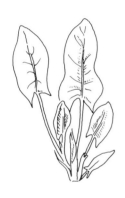

SORREL

It is rich in iron and in the oxalate of potash which give the leaves their sharp taste. It stimulates the appetite, provides energy, aids digestion, acts as a diuretic and can combat vitamin deficiencies. The leaves may be eaten raw in salads, while the soup (see page 255) is said to be as effective as the infusion: 1 oz. (30 g.) fresh or dried leaves to $1\frac{3}{4}$ pints (1 l.) boiling water, steeped for 10 minutes; take up to 3 wineglasses a day, but do not exceed this. It is also prescribed for high fevers – to quench thirst and lower the temperature – for haemorrhages and urinary disorders; it is good for the blood, especially as a spring strengthener. A cautionary word – the oxalic salts are not suitable to all conditions, and should not be taken by those suffering from gout, rheumatism, kidney stones or any lung disease, including asthma. The juice or infusion is used for ulcers in the mouth. Externally a poultice of cooked sorrel leaves will help abscesses, boils and sebaceous cysts. An infusion of $\frac{1}{2}$ cup to a quart (1 l.) of water can be used as a compress for cold sores.

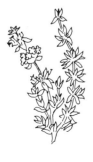

THYME

Garden thyme and wild thyme have the same effect; it is the essential oil that contains the medicinal qualities. It is a strong antiseptic, a stimulant for digestive, circulatory and respiratory systems. It also revives the nerve centres, and is a protection against catching colds and flu. An infusion is made from 1 oz. (30 g.) of the flowering tops (fresh or dried) to 1¾ pints (1 l.) of boiling water, steep for 10 minutes; take 3 – 4 wineglasses a day after or between meals. This tea can counteract drunkenness; a tea consisting of equal parts thyme and rosemary is a sound remedy for headaches and nervous problems. Coughs, catarrh and whooping cough can be helped by a strong infusion: 1 oz. (30 g.) to 18 fl. oz. (5 dl.) water, sweeten with honey; take 1 tablespoon five times a day. For an alternative cough medicine boil 1 tablespoon of whole linseed in 1¾ pints (1 l.) water for 5 minutes, pour this over 1 oz. (30 g.) thyme and a sliced lemon; sweeten with honey, stir well and strain when cold; take a tablespoonful five times a day.

Externally, an infusion of 2 oz. to a quart of water (50 g. to 1 l. water) is a gargle for sore throats and tonsillitis. It is a dependable disinfectant, preventing festering of cuts and gashes. A decoction of 1 lb. boiled in 6 pints water (500 g. in 4 l. water) for 5 minutes can be added to the bath water to stimulate circulation and help skin conditions; it eases rheumatism and arthritis too, though the oil essence of thyme is considered superior for this purpose – a few drops in the bath. Chopped thyme makes a good poultice for rheumatism. The powdered dried leaves, taken like snuff, will clear the nasal tract and stop nose bleeds.

VALERIAN

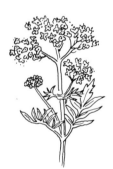

Only the root is used and it has a very sedative effect on the higher nerve centres. It is about the best herb for any nervous ailment and is used to benefit heart disorders of nervous origin, general agitation, overstrain and breakdowns – it causes none of the after-effects produced by narcotics. It allays pain and induces sleep; a tisane can cure congestion in the head, giddiness and fainting and ease headaches. Infuse a teaspoon of the crushed root in a cup of boiling water; take in small doses, a mouthful at a time, but no more than a cup a day. It is dangerous to mix it with orthodox drugs when used for insomnia.

NATURAL AIDS FOR DISEASES

Natural remedies can be used with advantage in healing; in some cases they are supportive only, while in others they are of vital significance. This chart will help you find which vegetable, fruit, herb or essence may be helpful in treating specific problems; for further details refer to the earlier chapters in this section where the remedies are described under the individual plants. Minor disorders may be treated at home, but before taking large quantities for long periods or for serious ailments professional advice must be sought.

ABSCESS

sunlight or other ultraviolet light; cabbage, cucumber and carrot juice; onion, leek, lettuce, fig, sorrel; agrimony tea; compresses of comfrey or marshmallow leaves; essential oils of bergamot or lavender.

ACNE

sunlight and fresh air; cabbage and tomato juice; turnip, lettuce and dandelion; dandelion or nettle tea; essential oils of bergamot, camphor, juniper or sandalwood.

ALCOHOLISM

fresh fruit and vegetable juices, particularly cabbage and parsley; brewer's yeast; thyme or fennel tea; essential oils of fennel or rose.

ANAEMIA

vegetable juices high in chlorophyll – spinach, cabbage, watercress, parsley, dandelion, seaweeds, bean, chicory; fruit juices – apricot, apple, black currant, black grape; herb teas – parsley, nettle; essential oil of camomile.

ARTERIOSCLEROSIS

vegetable juices – cabbage, carrot, tomato; fruit juices –

grapefruit, pineapple, lemon, apple; globe artichoke, garlic, cherry, plum; brewer's yeast; essential oils of juniper or rosemary.

ARTHRITIS (rheumatism)

vegetable juices – carrot, celery, red beet and, particularly, potato; fruit juices – pineapple and black currant; apple, globe artichoke, asparagus, radish, sorrel; herbal teas – nettle, sage, parsley, burdock root, peppermint; essential oils of camphor, eucalyptus, lavender, or rosemary for external massage.

ASTHMA

juices of garlic and horse-radish in small amounts mixed with vegetable juices of carrot and red beet; fruit juices – lime or lemon diluted in water; herbal teas – agrimony, marjoram, valerian root, camomile; essences of benzoin, eucalyptus, lavender, peppermint.

BITES

cabbage leaves; parsley juice; onion slices; herbal tea of fennel seed; crushed basil leaves.

BOILS

vegetable juice – carrot and

beet; tisane of nettle; essential oils of camomile or lavender, externally applied.

BRONCHITIS

lemon juice; onions, garlic, asparagus, cabbage, horse-radish, apple; mullein tea; inhalation from hot catnip tea; essential oils of benzoin, bergamot, camphor, cardamom, eucalyptus, lavender.

BRUISES

compress of comfrey; witch hazel massage; essential oils of camphor or hyssop.

BURNS

cabbage, potato applications; compresses of comfrey, elder flowers or marigold flowers; essential oils of peppermint, camomile, camphor; lavender, rosemary.

CATARRH

lemon juice and honey; onions and garlic; herbal teas of sage, elder flowers mixed with equal parts of peppermint and yarrow; mustard footbath; essential oils of eucalyptus, lavender or sandalwood as inhalations.

COLDS

vegetable juices – carrot, beet, green pepper, watercress, plus onion and garlic juice added in small doses, cabbage, orange; fruit juices – lemon, black currant, orange, elderberries; herbal teas – camomile, peppermint, lemon balm, sage; essential oils of camphor, eucalyptus, peppermint and rosemary.

COLIC

cucumber juice; herbal teas – camomile, peppermint with honey, thyme; essential oils of benzoin, bergamot, camomile, camphor, juniper, lavender.

COLITIS

cabbage juice; papaya juice; essential oils of bergamot, lavender, orange blossom.

CONSTIPATION

vegetable juices – spinach, watercress, nettles, dandelion, cucumber, cabbage, red beets; fruit juices – apples, lemon; herbal teas – dandelion, raspberry, parsley; essential oils of camphor, fennel, marjoram, rose.

CRAMPS

vegetable juices – carrot, beet, cucumber; sweet fruit juices; herbal teas – dandelion, thyme; essential oil of cloves as a massage.

DIABETES

vegetable juices – string beans, cabbage, parsley, cucumber, watercress; onion and garlic; citrus juices; string beans, cucumber, garlic; herbal teas – pods of string beans, dandelion roots, raspberry leaves; essential oils of eucalyptus, geranium and juniper.

DIARRHOEA

vegetable juice – cabbage, carrot, nettle; apricot, spinach, banana, papaya; herbal teas – blueberry, peppermint, raspberry leaf; essential oils of camomile, camphor, geranium, eucalyptus, lavender, orange blossom.

DIGESTIVE DISORDERS

vegetable juices – carrot, beet, celery, spinach; artichoke, fennel, parsley; fruit juices – papaya, apple, lemon, pineapple; herbal teas – camomile, peppermint, thyme, parsley; essential oils of bergamot, cardamom, orange blossom, rosemary.

ECZEMA

juices of green vegetables, particularly spinach, also cucumber, carrot, beet, celery; watercress, spinach, raw potatoes; fruit juices – black currant, lemon; herbal teas of marigold, burdock, strawberry leaves; essential oils of lavender, juniper, bergamot.

FEVER

fruit juices – lemon or grapefruit; herbal teas – yarrow, marigold flowers; essential oils of bergamot, eucalyptus, camphor.

GALL BLADDER PROBLEMS

vegetable juices – beet tops, cabbage, small amounts of dandelion or radish; fruit juices – pear, lemon, grapefruit, grape; herbal teas – dandelion, fennel, parsley; essential oils of bergamot, lavender, rosemary.

GOUT

vegetable juices – carrot, celery, potato; pears, cherries; pineapple juice; herbal teas – juniper berries, parsley; essential oils of benzoin, camphor, juniper.

HAEMORRHOIDS

vegetable juices – cabbage, potato; dandelion leaf; fruit juices – lemon, orange, papaya, pineapple, grapefruit; herbal teas of yarrow, rose hips; suppositories – raw garlic clove, raw potato; essential oil of juniper.

HALITOSIS

all green vegetable juices; parsley; herbal teas – parsley, peppermint, rosemary; essential oils of bergamot, lavender, cardamom.

HEADACHES

cabbage juice; apple juice;

herbal infusions – mint, camomile, lemon balm; essential oils of cardamom, lavender, rose.

HEART DISEASE

vegetable juices – carrot, asparagus, beet, celery; watercress, parsley; fruit juices – black currant, rose hip, blueberry; herbal teas – valerian root, hawthorn leaves, rosemary; essential oils of camphor, lavender, rose, orange blossom.

HIGH BLOOD PRESSURE

vegetable juices – carrots, spinach, beet, parsley, small amounts of garlic; fruit juices – all citrus fruits, black currant, grape; herbal tea – valerian root; essential oil of lavender.

INSOMNIA

lettuce; herbal teas – valerian, lettuce; essential oils of orange blossom, rose, sandalwood, lavender.

KIDNEY DISORDERS

vegetable juices – cucumber, celery, carrots; horse-radish, watercress, garlic, grapes; fruit juices – water-melon, lemon, orange; herbal teas – dandelion, parsley; essential oils of eucalyptus, juniper, sandalwood.

LARYNGITIS

vegetable juices – cabbage, celery; garlic, raw onions, fig, fresh fruits; fruit juices – lemon, apple; herbal teas – sage, nettle, yarrow; essential oils of benzoin, lavender, sandalwood.

LIVER PROBLEMS

vegetable juices – red beet with small amounts of radish, artichoke, asparagus, cabbage, dandelion; fruit juices – grape, lemon, papaya; herbal teas – dandelion, parsley; essential oils of lavender, juniper, geranium, rose.

MENOPAUSE

vegetable juices – artichoke, cabbage, carrot, spinach; fruit juices – cherry, apricot, orange; herbal teas – elder flowers, peppermint; essential oils of fennel, camomile.

MENSTRUAL DISORDERS

all green vegetable juices, red beet, lettuce; fennel, fig, parsley; fruit juices – grape, black currant; herbal teas – parsley, yarrow, mint; essential oils of rose, juniper, lavender, mint.

NAUSEA

peppermint tea; essential oils of lavender, cardamom.

NERVOUS COMPLAINTS

vegetable juices – beet, cabbage, celery; apricot, avocado, celery, aubergine; fruit juices – apple, peach, pineapple; herbal teas – basil, sage, valerian, rosemary, marjoram; essential oils of benzoin, bergamot, geranium, jasmine, lavender, rose, sandalwood.

OEDEMA (excessive fluid retention)

vegetable juices – cucumber, garlic, celery; cabbage, fennel, parsley, grape; fruit juices – pineapple, water-melon; herbal teas – juniper berries, parsley; essential oils of benzoin, camphor, geranium, juniper.

RHEUMATISM (*see* Arthritis)

SENILITY

vegetable juices – cabbage, carrot, spinach; artichoke, garlic, seaweeds, apricots, date, fig; fruit juices – pineapple, papaya, lemon; herbal teas – elder flowers, ginseng; essential oils of jasmine, lavender, rose.

STOMACH ULCERS

vegetable juices – potato, cabbage; herbal teas – violet, cloves, camomile; essential oils of camomile, geranium.

URINARY TRACT INFECTIONS

vegetable juices – cabbage, watercress; dandelion, lettuce, chicory; essential oils of bergamot, eucalyptus, juniper, lavender.

WOUNDS

vegetable juices – cabbage, celery, parsley; compresses – cabbage or comfrey; essential oils of bergamot, camphor, geranium, juniper, lavender, rosemary.

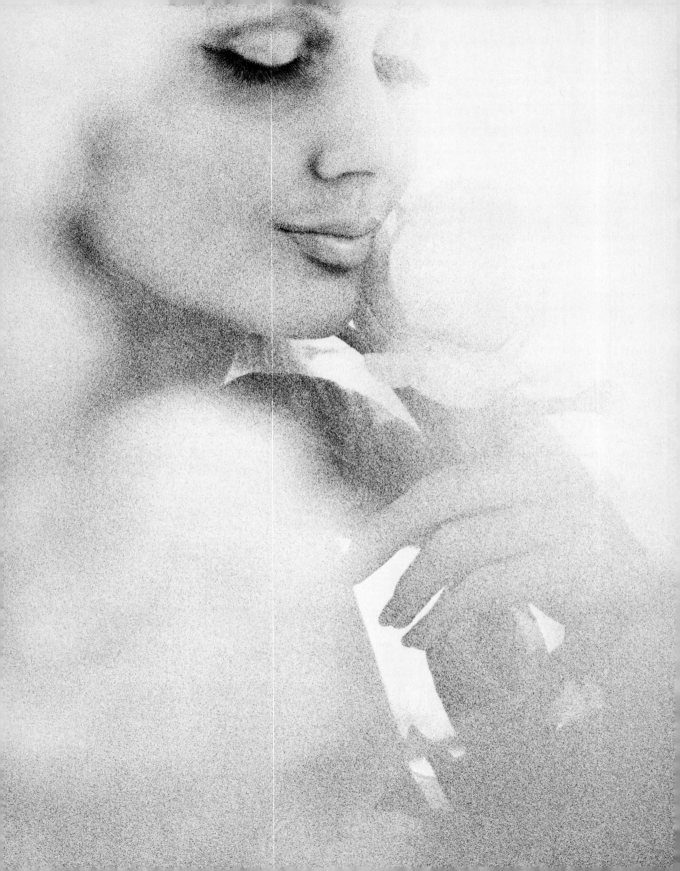

3

ESSENCES AND FLOWERS

Healing by means of aromatic flowers is an ancient art that is now used in two ways: through remedies prepared by immersing flowers in water, the essenced liquid being potentized – diluted to an infinitesimal degree – and taken orally; or by treating the body with the essential oils of flowers and plants, both externally and internally. The first method is the original creation of Dr Edward Bach, a British physician who pioneered a new way of flower healing during the 1920s and 1930s. The other method is known as aromatherapy, and, though very important in old Chinese and Indian medicine, it has only recently come into its own again through research over the past forty years. The protagonist of modern aromatherapy was René-Maurice Gattefossé, a French doctor, who published a comprehensive book on the subject in the late 1920s. More recently another Frenchman, Jean Valnet, has contributed most to the medical assessment and acceptance of the treatment.

THE BACH FLOWER REMEDIES

These are unusual in that they are prescribed not directly for a biological complaint but according to moods and personality traits, expressed in fear, worry, anger or depression. Dr Bach considered that an inharmonious state of mind caused sickness and disease and that it also slowed recovery. The idea that a flower can help the mind to cure the body sounds improbable, yet over the years the remedies have proved to be extremely effective. The treatment is based on the principle of helping the body to achieve its optimum state of positive thinking, vitality and peace in order to restore health through its own biological powers. In treating cases, the Bach theory (currently practised by many naturopathic doctors) is to disregard the disease itself; the outlook of the patient is the guide to which remedy or remedies are necessary. Dr Bach always stressed that his remedies could be used in conjunction with any other form of treatment as they would not clash or interfere with other régimes. The flower remedies are significant prevention measures, harmless in themselves, yet capable of conveying a forceful energy pattern which is considered to be the vital issue in any nature healing.

Dr Bach believed that help for the body through nature was within reach of everyone. He selected the flowers instinctively and tested them on himself in the standard homoeopathic way. He was the first to show that the healing power of plants can be transmitted to water by immersion alone.

The remedies are said never to produce an unpleasant reaction and can be safely prescribed and used by anyone. Self-treatment requires sensitive observation of personal reactions particularly when tired, under stress, during a crisis of worry, fear or indecision.

The Bach Centre in Sotwell, Oxfordshire, carries on Dr Bach's work of advice and preparation of the remedies, which are also obtainable at certain specialized chemists. Preparation is extraordinarily simple and can be done by anyone. It incorporates the essentials of nature, the four elements of earth, air, fire and water: earth where the flowers grew, air surrounding them during the potentizing process, fire from the sun, and water. A thin shallow glass bowl is filled with 1 pint (6 dl.) of the purest water possible (spring or well water is preferable; some municipal tap waters are adequate, but do not use distilled water). The flowers are gathered in full bloom, immediately floated on the water to cover the entire surface and left in bright sunshine for 3 to 4 hours, or less if the blossoms start to fade. This is a potent way of impregnating water with the 'virtue' of the flower. The liquid is poured into bottles mixed with equal parts of brandy. This is basic stock, which is further diluted, usually 5 drops to 1 fluid ounce (0·28 dl.) of water, from which the remedial dosage is 5 drops in a tablespoon of water to be taken two or three times a day. There is no chance of taking too much or too often, though the smallest quantities are capable of beneficial action. In urgent cases, a remedy can be taken every few minutes until there is improvement; in severe cases every half hour.

The remedies help the most common negative states of mind. They can be used singly or in combination, and it is interesting to note the correlation between many of these recommendations and those suggested by herbalists (see the chapter on herbs and tisanes, pages 117ff) particularly for disorders of nervous origin. The flowers are:

Agrimony: To help mental stress and worry, particularly when concealed from others beneath a veneer of gaiety.

Aspen: When fears, anxiety and apprehension are present, but their origin is unknown.

Beech: For intolerant natures, prone to criticizing others and passing judgements.

Centaury: Weak-willed characters, too easily influenced by others and too eager to serve.

Cerato: Self-doubt, foolishness.

Cherry-plum: For a fear of losing control, a dread of doing something awful.

Chestnut bud: Failure to learn by experience.

Chicory: Possessiveness, self-love and self-pity.

Clematis: Indifference to reality, dreaminess and inattention.

Crab apple: For despondency and despair.

Elm (Ulmus procra): For those who strive too hard for perfection, resulting in exhaustion, despondency and feelings of inadequacy.

Gentian: Helps doubt, depression and discouragement.

Gorse: For when feelings of despair amount to hopelessness.

Heather: For the self-centred.

Holly: Combats jealousy, envy, suspicion and hatred.

Honeysuckle: Living in the past, nostalgia and homesickness.

Hornbeam: For general tiredness, physical and mental exhaustion.

Impatiens: When extreme mental tension leads to utter impatience and irritability.

Larch: Lack of confidence, anticipation of failure, despondency.

Mimulus: Calms in the case of a fear or anxiety of known origin.

Mustard: For depression and gloom.

Oak: When despondency and despair is accompanied with effort to counteract it.

Olive: Complete exhaustion and mental fatigue.

Pine: To help balance feelings of guilt and self-reproach leading to despondency.

Red chestnut: When excessive fear is mainly anxiety for others.

Rock rose: To counteract fright, panic and terror.

Rock water: For those who deny and repress themselves, self-martyrdom.
Scleranthus: Uncertainty, indecision, imbalance and hesitancy.
Sweet chestnut: An aid for extreme mental anguish and despair.
Vervain: For stress, strain and tension.
Vine: For dominating people with inflexible ambitions.
Walnut: For those oversensitive to ideas and influences.
Water violet: Pride, aloofness.
White chestnut: For a mind full of unwanted thoughts, mental arguments and conversations.
Wild oat: Uncertainty, dissatisfaction and despondency.
Wild rose: For apathy.
Willow: Bitterness and resentment.

AROMATIC TREATMENT WITH ESSENCES

Plant essences have been compared to blood; they are not the entire plant but they are complete in themselves and like blood they contain the elements and characteristics of the plant from which they come. The essence is the most ethereal part and its therapeutic agents act more on the mind and emotions than do other herbal treatments. In this, the aromatic method of healing bears a relation to the flower remedies. The properties of herbs and their essences may be the same, but their influence on the body is often different.

They have a consistency more like water than oil; most are clear though some are coloured. Their chemistry is complex, but they are soluble in alcohol, ether and fixed oils, and partially soluble in water. A mixture of essential oil and water is often the best medium for energy vibrations. Water appears to have a catalytic effect on the essences, drawing out their power in a beneficial way. Baths perfumed with aromatics are recommended for various ailments and noteworthy results are claimed for simple foot baths.

Aromatherapy involves external and internal treatments; the professional practitioner prescribes a combination of aromatics in all applications – massage, inhalation and oral. Essential oils can be absorbed by the body through the skin and rapidly penetrate organs via the nervous system and sometimes the endocrine system. They are capable of stimulating and healing internal metabolisms and muscles. They do not act by a chemical procedure, but by energy and radiation. The odorous molecule possesses a greater number of free electrons than a normal organic molecule, and this gives off special power. The oil does not remain in the body; having induced biological action it is eliminated through the lungs, the urine and the skin.

At home one can benefit from essences by means of bathing, douches, inhalations, massaging and, to some extent, by oral intake.

Baths

Because many oils only partially dissolve in water, it is important to fill the bath (warm water) first and then drop in oils. On average, 5 or 6 drops are needed, but this varies and you may require as few as 2 or up to 10. Start with a small amount and progressively add more – but remember the benefits are subtle and not immediately apparent. Here are some baths to try for certain effects; the number of drops recommended are in brackets.

Relaxing bath: Lavender (5), cypress (5), marjoram (4), camomile (2), orange blossom (2), rose (2).

Stimulating bath: Rosemary (5), juniper (5), hyssop (3), peppermint (3), basil (3).

Refreshing bath: Lavender (5), juniper (5), cypress (5), geranium (4), lemon (4), peppermint (4), bergamot (3).

Sensual bath: Sandalwood (8), ylang-ylang (3), orange blossom (2), jasmine (2).

Some special baths require a combination of oils; the proportions are delicately balanced and the number of drops, given in parenthesis, should not be altered:

For nervous exhaustion: Basil (2), geranium (4) and hyssop (2).
Sedative bath: Camomile (2), lavender (5) and orange blossom (2).
To give morning energy: Rosemary (5), juniper (5) and peppermint (2).
For winter rawness: Juniper (3), pepper (2) and lavender (5).
For a hangover: Fennel (2), rosemary (2) and juniper (4).

Douches

Use 5 to 10 drops in combination to 2 pints (1 l.) water.
For painful periods: Clary (4), marjoram (3), and peppermint (2).
For leucorrhoea: Bergamot (2), lavender (4) and rose (2).

Inhalations

Six to 12 drops in combination in a bowl of steaming water.

    For congested head cold: Eucalyptus (6), peppermint (2) and basil (2).

    For influenza: Eucalyptus (7), camphor (3) and black pepper (2).

    For bronchitis: Eucalyptus (4), bergamot orange (4) and sandalwood (4).

    For asthma and bronchitis: Lavender (6), hyssop (3) and peppermint (3).

Massages

Use 10 to 30 drops per oz. (30 g.) distributing oil.

    For muscles and aches: Juniper (10), lavender (5) and rosemary (5) mixed in a vegetable oil in a dilution of 3 per cent.

    For rheumatic pain: Eucalyptus (7), camphor (7) and rosemary (7) combined in a vegetable oil in a dilution of 5 per cent.

    To bring general relaxation: Geranium (10), lavender (5) and marjoram (4) in an oil dilution of 2 per cent.

    To arouse sensuality: Sandalwood (7), bergamot (7), jasmine (3) and rose (3), in an oil dilution of 2 per cent.

Oral Medicines

Each prescription should be taken three times a day (the number of drops is given in parenthesis) in sweetened water.

    For indigestion: Basil (1), juniper (2), peppermint (1) and cardamon (1).

    For coughs: Hyssop (3), cypress (2), and lavender (2).

    For gall stones: Rosemary (2), bergamot (2) and eucalyptus (1).

The Bach remedies and aromatherapy together provide the major part of benefit from flowers and essences, though some can be made into simple teas and compresses, tinctures and ointments. The following is a list of the more important flowers and essences, together with their properties and use.

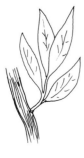

BENZOIN

This is a tree cultivated in the Far East, and the essence comes from the gum formed when a deep incision is made in the trunk. It is commonly known as friar's balsam and is a traditional inhalant for head colds and any sinus blockage. It is useful for all cold conditions related to the respiratory tract – coughs, asthma, bronchitis and influenza. It can be taken internally – 3 drops three times a day in sweetened water – or in inhalations, where 6 to 12 drops are put in boiling water for steaming. It is also helpful in conditions of the urinary system and can be used for cystitis. Externally it can aid skin problems such as irritation or itching, dry cracked skin and wounds. A massage oil will relieve joints afflicted with gout and rheumatism.

CLOVES

The undeveloped flowers give out their oil when simply squeezed with the fingernail. Clove stalks can be taken in powder form or as an infusion for nausea and indigestion. A tea made from a mixture of cloves, allspice, ginger and cinnamon, infused with a little brandy and left to warm in the sun, can help to relieve colic. Clove oil is extremely stimulating; it is antiseptic and a painkiller, and is frequently used for toothache and to clear bronchial blockages.

DAISY

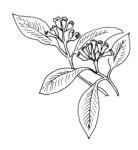

It is the ox-eye daisy that is used medically; this is taller than the common daisy and is often known as a marguerite. The flowers are balsamic; an infusion will relieve coughs and catarrhs – boil flowers, leaves and stalks together and sweeten with honey. Used externally it has been successfully used in healing wounds, as a poultice or an infusion mixed with lard or lanolin for an ointment.

DANDELION

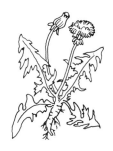
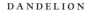

A particularly valuable plant – all parts are beneficial. The young leaves are a concentrated source of vitamin A, and a good source of vitamins B and C. The leaves can be eaten raw in a salad, cooked like spinach or made into a broth or tea; they act as a prime blood cleanser and an aid to digestion, benefiting the kidneys, liver and gall bladder. All parts of the plant contain a healthful juice, latex, but for healing the most powerful part is the root: boil 2 oz. (60 g.) freshly sliced root in 2 pints (1 l.) water, until reduced to 1 pint (6 dl.) and add 1 oz. (30 g.) compound tincture of horse-radish –

particularly aids a sluggish liver given in daily doses of 2–4 oz. (60–120 g.). The flowers are used to make a tea for rheumatic and related problems: pour a pint (6 dl.) boiling water on 1 oz. (30 g.) flowers. Dandelion flowers also make an excellent tonic wine, reputed to be good for the blood: pour 1 gallon (4·5 l.) boiling water over 1 gallon (4·5 l.) of flowers; stir well, cover with a porous cloth and allow to stand for 3 days, stirring every now and then; strain; add 3 lb. (1·4 kg.) sugar, a little sliced ginger, the rind of a lemon and orange (sliced, not grated) and boil for 30 minutes; allow to cool; put a little yeast on a piece of toast, float on the liquid; cover and stand for 2 days; bottle and keep for 2 months before use.

EUCALYPTUS

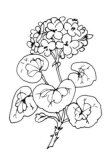

The essential oil comes from the leaves and was once considered a general cure-all. It has an impressive history as an inhalant or chest rub, and today is probably best known for its value in most respiratory disorders including sinusitis and tuberculosis. It has a definite cooling effect on the body and is capable of bringing about a marked decrease in temperature – because of this it is prescribed for malaria, typhus, measles and influenza. It is an effective antiseptic oil, and it is good used externally for skin eruptions, including herpes. Massaged into affected areas, it helps muscular or rheumatic pain and can be applied continuously for rheumatoid arthritis.

GERANIUM

The entire plant is aromatic and the essence is relaxing and refreshing. Its action on the nervous system is of particular significance as it is both calming and uplifting; it is used to treat anxiety and depression, and pain of a nervous origin. It can also influence the hormone system and help bring about a balance in the secretion of androgen and oestrogen, which often becomes irregular during the menopause. It is a mild diuretic and used internally for stones of the urinary passages. Externally, it aids wounds, burns and ulcers. It is one of the best skin-care agents, cleansing, refreshing and nourishing, especially for oily skin.

JASMINE

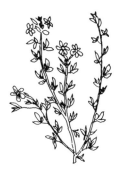

The essence comes from the flowers and is given for psychological and psychosomatic problems. Although it has specific physical benefits, it is thought to be more effective when these are bound to an emotional state. It is an anti-depressant and gives a feeling of optimism and confidence; it is a nerve sedative which is also uplifting, and is therefore useful in cases of apathy and listlessness. The oil influences the respiratory tract, aiding coughs, hoarseness, laboured breathing and bronchial difficulties. It can strengthen a weak stomach. Of particular interest to women is its action on the female reproductive system – it can help menstrual pains in the stomach or the back, it lessens the pain of delivery and accelerates birth, it aids the milk flow and can be used externally as a massage oil on stomach skin after birth. A syrup prepared from the fresh flowers is good for bronchial disorders: an infusion of 6 oz. flowers to 1 quart boiling water (150 g. flowers to 1 l. water), strain, add honey and boil to make a syrup.

JUNIPER

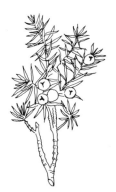

The berries provide the essence. It is a traditional aid for urinary infections, acting as a diuretic. It is of value in cases of cystitis and kidney stones. Its water-emitting action also makes it a suitable remedy for gout and rheumatism. It can be used for indigestion and related stomach problems, for colic and flatulence. It is an antiseptic for the blood and stimulates circulation, thereby aiding skin troubles. It helps counteract stress and anxiety, and when used in a bath before going to bed its calming action will induce sleep. Externally, it can be applied for skin irritations.

LAVENDER

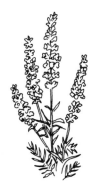

This is considered the most useful and versatile of the essential oils; the essence comes from the flowers, which can be used to make teas and infusions of considerable therapeutic value. Lavender is, of course, notable for its delicious smell, which is refreshing; it calms and can help nervous and psychological disorders including depression, nervous tension, migraine and insomnia. A lavender bath can be very soothing to an overactive brain: put 6 drops of lavender oil in a warm bath, or boil a handful of flowers for 10 minutes, strain, and add to the bath water. To further this calming treatment, sprinkle a few drops of lavender essence on the pillow – deep, regular breaths of this aromatic induce sleep. This sedative action can also help palpitations, lower high blood pressure and counterbalance the agitation from nervous exhaustion. Digestive disorders associated with nervous or emotional problems are relieved – colic, nausea, vomiting and flatulence. It also encourages appetite. A few drops of lavender oil rubbed on the temple will alleviate a nervous headache and mental depression. A tea brewed from a half-cupful of lavender flowers to a pint (6 dl.) of boiling water, can be sipped to relieve headaches due to tiredness. A few drops of the essence in a footbath will help general fatigue. The oil is also useful in many aspects of childbirth, having a calming effect and helping to hasten delivery. It is a good remedy for sunstroke. Externally, lavender oil can stimulate paralysed limbs; mixed with $\frac{3}{4}$ spirit of turpentine it helps sprains and stiff joints. Milder solutions (less than 1 per cent in other oils or fats) aid skin conditions, though it is often better to combine it with camomile.

MARIGOLD

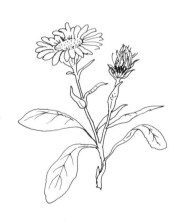

It is only the common deep-orange-flowered variety that is of medicinal value. Flowers should be used fresh or quickly dried in the shade. It is a basic healing flower that encourages the making of healthy tissue. The infusion of 1 oz. (30 g.) to a pint (6 dl.) of boiling water is given internally in doses of a tablespoonful three or four times a day; a milder tisane is made from 1 oz. (30 g.) of the flowers to 2 pints (1 l.) water, and 3 or 4 cupfuls may be taken daily. It is recommended to prevent inflammation and promote healing in cases of gastritis, enteritis and ulcers; it can relieve congestion in liver complaints and may be used as a treatment for menopausal disorders and irregular or painful menstruation – for the latter, treatment should begin a week before the period is due. It is said to prevent continued vomiting. If the tea is taken after an accident, it brings out bruises and helps prevent internal complications. The constant use of the tea can balance nervous disorders and help skin problems. Externally, an infusion in compress form assists in the healing of burns, relieves the pain and prevents the formation of scars. Fresh flowers, chopped up, can be applied too. Petals soaked in oil help heal old wounds and scars. They are said to be one of the best treatments for chilblains: soak for a long time in a basin containing 3oz. (90g.) flowers to 2 pints (1l.) water warmed to 98°F (37°C); afterwards cover the afflicted parts with a poultice of the boiled flowers.

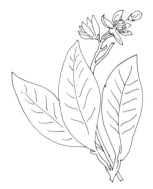

ORANGE BLOSSOM

The essence from the flowers is one of the most effective anti-depressant aromatics. It calms and slows down the mind, and is particularly helpful for people who panic and become irrationally distressed. It is used for palpitations and other cardiac spasms, or when disorders or agitation cause strain on the heart. It is valuable in cases of shock: a bath containing 6 drops of the essential oil is soothing and comforting; at the same time it helps the skin as it encourages the shedding of old cells and the growth of new. In particular it aids dry skin and broken veins.

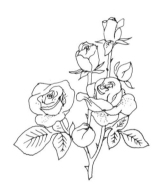

ROSE

This is the least toxic of all the essences and has many healing and beneficial qualities. Its most important action is its influence on the circulatory system – it promotes circulation, relieves heart congestion, tones the capillaries and cleanses the blood. It strengthens the stomach and facilitates the elimination process. It has a calming control over the nerves, and can be used as an anti-depressant. Indeed the overall action is particularly suited to helping cases of stress and tension. A vinegar made from roses is good for headaches caused by the sun – compresses are applied to the forehead. An infusion of dried petals (2 oz. to a quart of boiling water – 50 g. to a litre – infused for 15 minutes) is a lotion for compresses to help conjunctivitis.

Rose honey is an old remedy for sore throats and inflammation of the mucous membranes: boil 1 oz. (30 g.) of rose petals in 3½ oz. (100 g.) honey for 10 minutes, press and strain. Externally rose oil helps all skins because of its action on the capillaries.

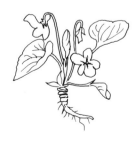

VIOLET, SWEET

The flowers are used to make syrup of violets which acts as a pleasant laxative and is helpful to the kidneys: to 1 lb. fresh flowers add 2½ pints boiling water (500 g. flowers to 1·5 l. water), infuse for 24 hours; pour off the liquid, strain; then, using double its weight in sugar, heat to form a syrup, but do not bring to the boil. A flower tea helps cold and bronchitis sufferers: pour ½ pint (3 dl.) boiling water on to 1 teaspoon dried violets; cover and infuse for 5 minutes; sweeten with honey. Poultices of the leaves or flowers can be applied to swellings and inflammations.

AIR AND
EARTH

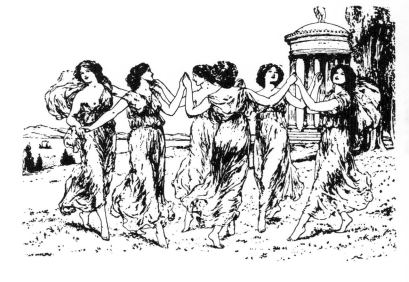

Right, *'Out of health beauty is created, and only by good health can beauty live.*
St Ivel Lactic Cheese is the ideal health food. It contains an abundance of natural properties which nourish and feed the body, without overheating the blood or taxing the digestion.'

Beauty and Health go hand in hand

1916

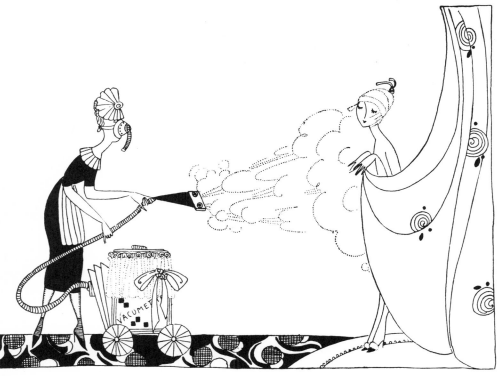

Left, LEADING THE SIMPLE LIFE IN LONDON
'There are even delicate rumours about the use of the "de-fardeur", so extraordinary an accessory for the boudoir, yet doubtless quite necessary in these days of smoke and powder.'

FISH 1920

Right, SMART LIFE BY THE OCEAN WAVES
'No wonder the beaches are popular! Where else would one wear a costume of seagreen duvetine under a cape of gay rubberized silk, or a bathing-suit of white foulard dotted and bound with bright red? The coat of white polo cloth has pipings of black, coral, and yellow.'

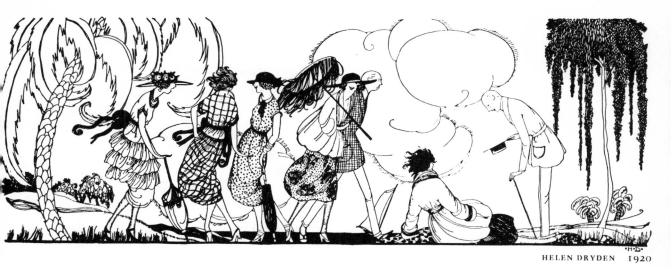

HELEN DRYDEN 1920

Above, *'Palm-trees and moss-hung live-oaks, tumbled clouds, and billowing sails, ruffles of organdie, ribbons, and parasols – all turned to gold by the sun's Midas fingers – that is the spell of the South.'*

Right, MATERIAL INDICATIONS OF A CHANGE OF CLIMATE
'Escorted by the large beach umbrella, the henna-coloured voile dress promises a successful morning besides the waves. Its white voile ruffles have scalloped henna-coloured edges. Overtunics of English silk in dull blue and green forget-me-nots, tie about the organdie frock in the middle with old-blue ribbons. Under the huge hat is a frock of pale grey Swiss with a plain grey organdie gilet and a bit of black ribbon.'

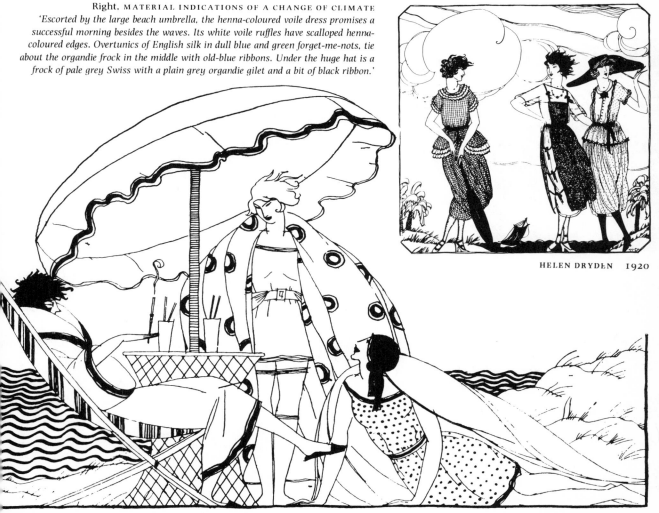

HELEN DRYDEN 1920

HELEN DRYDEN 1921

Right, BEAUTY BASED ON HEALTH
'In the ozone-filled room. sleep very soon descends upon the reader. To what extent will beauty be achieved under this régime? Perhaps all one's expectations will at last be fulfilled.'

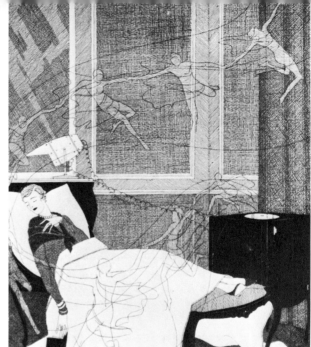

J. PAGES 1928

Below, VERVE 'Life gives one so much pleasure! So many places to amuse oneself, so many charming people to meet. Charm, allure, pleasure everywhere. You only need verve, warmth, gaiety and a svelte and gracious body. For this joie de vivre it is necessary to follow a series of Elizabeth Arden exercises.'

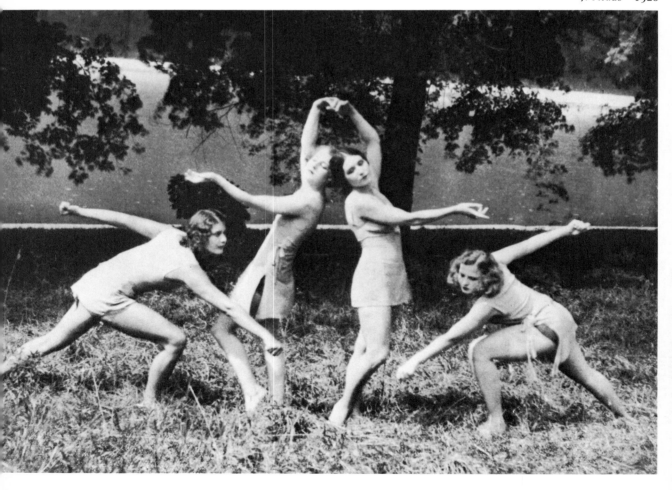

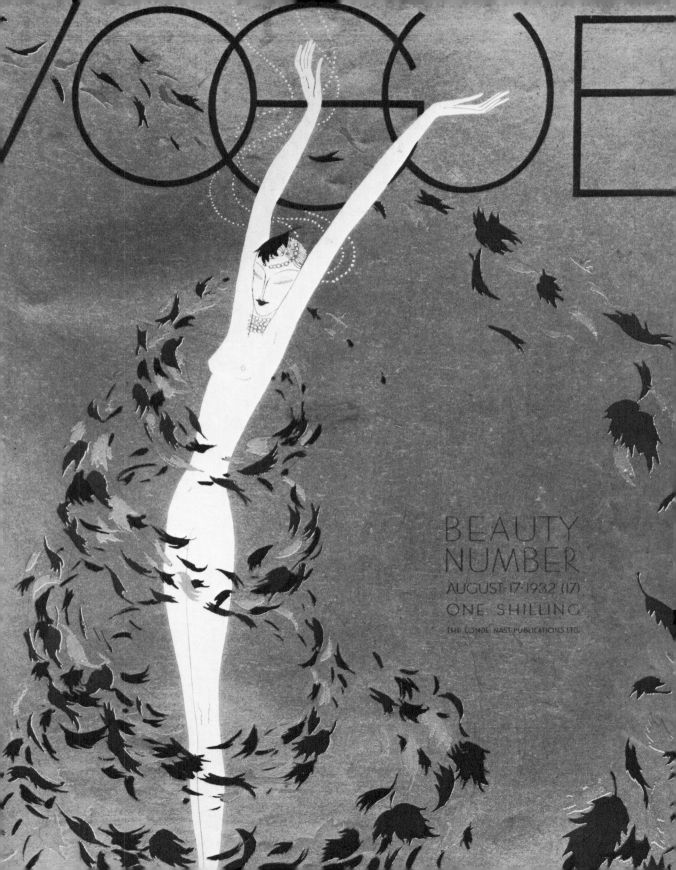

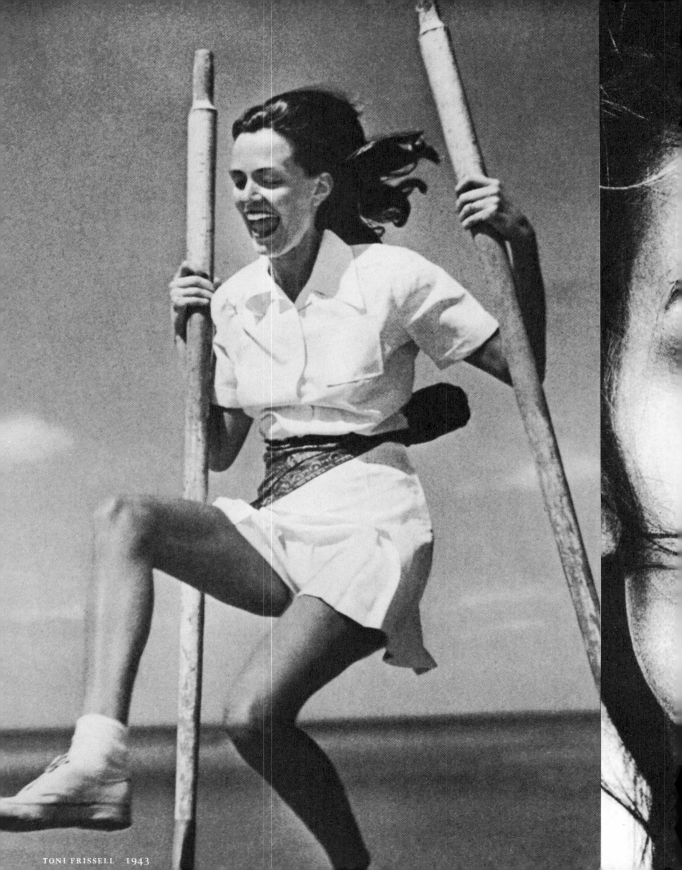

TONI FRISSELL 1943

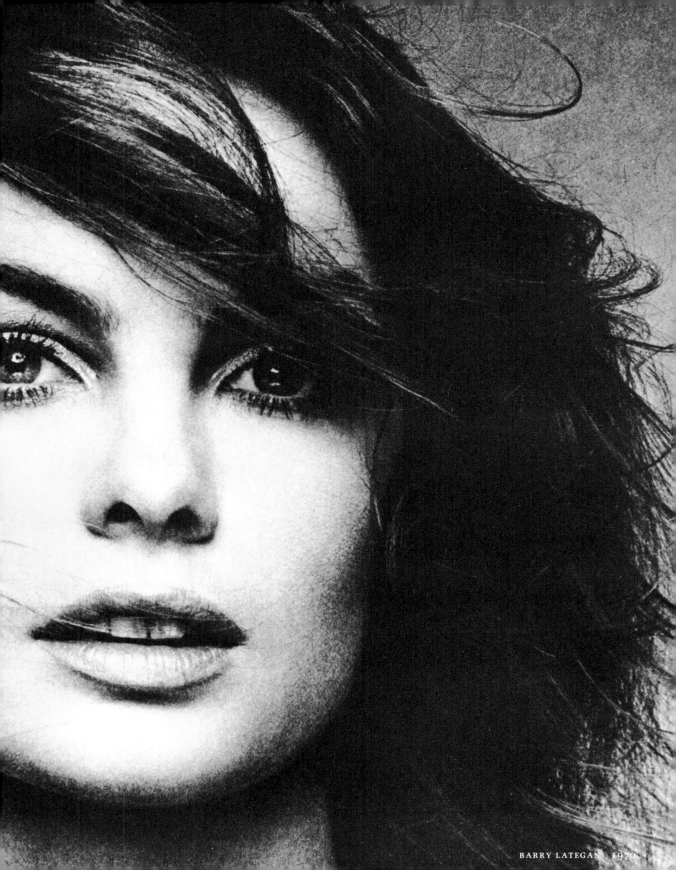

BARRY LATEGAN 1970

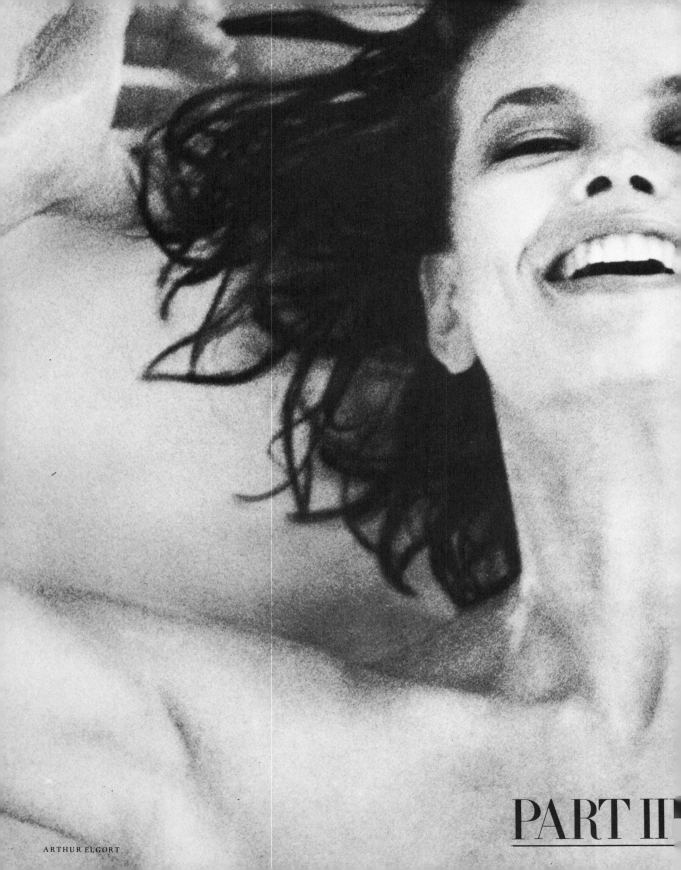

ARTHUR ELGORT

PART II

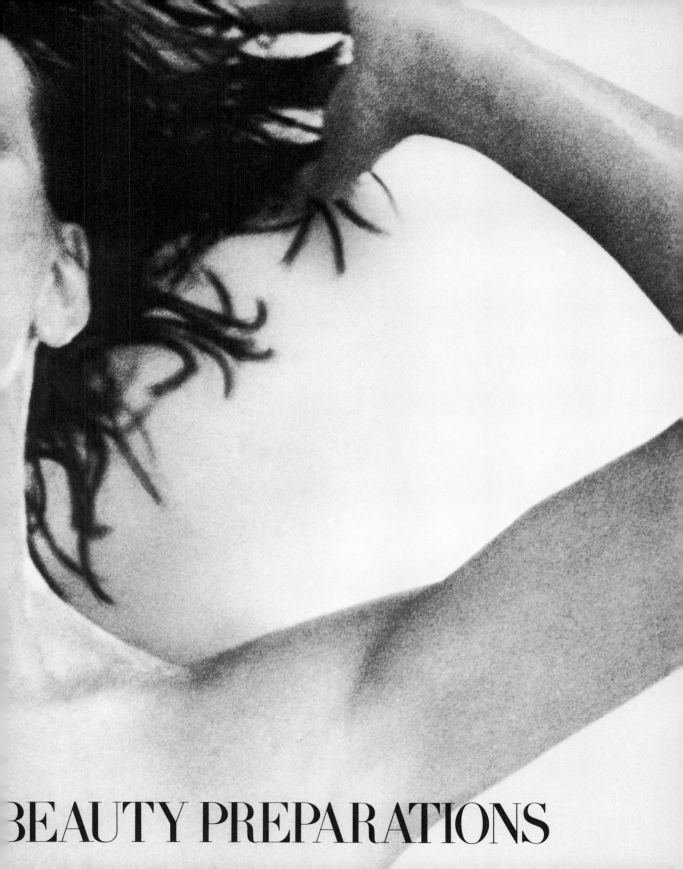

BEAUTY PREPARATIONS

Looking to nature for effective aids is becoming an accepted part of a beauty régime. Not that it is new; throughout history women have experimented with all kinds of plants, flowers and foods for cosmetic use. What is significant, however, is that over the past few years, the value of natural ingredients has been acknowledged. Old lore and recipes have been scientifically sifted and the fiction discarded. It must be pointed out that the nature part of beauty is to do with basic care and conditioning – primarily the health of skin and hair. The cosmetics of artifice – make-up, tints, polishes – are still the realm of the professional laboratory. But, given time and patience and practice, you can make many creams and lotions at home.

It is probable that cosmetics originated in China four thousand years ago, though herbal documents of that time dealt solely with the medicinal and culinary use of plants. The earliest evidence comes from Egypt, with records of kohl, henna, fragrant oils, mud and milk. The Romans developed bathing to a high degree of sophistication, but did little for cosmetics. Europe was very slow to develop beautifying creams or lotions because Christianity frowned upon vanity. The situation in the Middle East was quite different and over the years knowledge of oils and fragrances was accumulated; at the time of the Crusades many new ideas and potions were brought north.

In general, the preparations we know today began as hygienic aids to treat skin blemishes and rashes. In time they began to be used as preventive measures, finally as beautifying agents. In the sixteenth and seventeenth centuries herbalism was in its prime and resulted in books detailing recipes for health and beauty through plants, many based on Greek and Roman records – still the nucleus for today's prescriptions.

Most of the constructive aids and recipes have their origin in the nineteenth century, when the look of beauty changed from the powdered and brightly coloured face to one of pretty, natural delicacy. Cosmetics were made from flowers, herbs, plants and oils, and women were instructed how to make their own at home. These have been investigated in the light of modern knowledge, and adjusted and improved to fit today's needs.

Natural preparations are no miracle workers. There is an element of trial and error in the making and in the using. Not all recipes are suitable for everyone; it is a very flexible form of cosmetology and you need to learn to adjust ingredients and quantities for your individual needs and conditions. At least the risk of harm is negligible. Don't expect your products to look like commercial ones; don't expect them to last long either, as home-made treatments lack the usual commercial preservatives. The ingredients are readily available – the oils and fats from most druggists, the fragrant oils and dried herbs from a herbal supplier. Today many of the ingredients can also be obtained from health food stores.

Many of the following are simple one-product beauty aids; and the ingredients often common kitchen ones. The compounds are easy to formulate, but be sure to use glass, ceramic or enamel pots and containers and wooden spoons for stirring; the old-fashioned pestle and mortar is still the best way to grind grains, fresh and dried plants. For instructions on making an infusion see page 119. Anything that has perishable food in it has to be refrigerated.

1

SKIN

Good skin is achieved through constant care; it requires daily attention to cleansing, freshening, moisturizing and conditioning. The first three take only a few minutes in sequence, and ideally should be done twice daily. Conditioning creams can stay on overnight or alternatively for a couple of hours during the day. Weekly exfoliation (thinning to get rid of the dead cell build-up) and facial treatments stimulate and nourish the skin, helping to keep it in an active and healthy state. Natural applications give very satisfactory results, and there is a long list to choose from.

SKIN TREATMENT SCHEDULE

	OILY SKIN	DRY SKIN	BALANCED SKIN
Twice daily (morning and evening)	Cleanse with soap or cleanser, and water	Cleanse with soap, cream or lotion, and water	Cleanse with soap, cream or lotion, and water
	Astringent Light moisturizer	Freshener (toner) Rich moisturizer	Freshener (toner) Light moisturizer
Daily	Eye cream Conditioner for throat area	Eye cream Rich cream conditioner	Eye cream Light cream conditioner
Weekly	Exfoliation treatment (twice a week is better)	Exfoliation treatment (frequently if dry skin builds up)	Exfoliation treatment
Weekly	Stimulation and clearing facial	Stimulation and nourishing facial	Stimulation and clearing facial

CLEANSERS

There is no substitute for a good mild soap for cleansing the body (see page 187) and it is rare for a woman to be so sensitive to soap that she has to avoid it altogether. However, facial skin sometimes needs special attention, and the alternatives are particularly refreshing and often nourishing at the same time.

Simple Cleansers

Any vegetable oil will remove make-up, including the more obstinate eye colourings and mascara; simply put a little on a wad of cottonwool and gently clean. Almond oil and coconut oil are specially recommended. Other simple cleansers are fresh potato juice, strawberry juice, warm milk and natural yogurt; although these clean the skin admirably, they are not always so successful at clearing away the heavier make-up.

Recipes

Oatmeal Cleanser Using unprocessed oatmeal (not instant) grind to a powder and add enough cream or milk to make a fairly stiff paste. Rub on and into any particularly dirty area; rinse away.

Basic Light Cleansing Cream
$\frac{1}{2}$ oz. (15 g.) white wax
6 tablespoons almond oil
$\frac{1}{4}$ teaspoon boric acid powder
5 tablespoons distilled water

Melt the wax in a double boiler (or in a glass bowl inserted in simmering water) and slowly add the almond oil. In a separate dish dissolve the boric acid powder in the warmed distilled water; add this to the wax and oil; remove from the heat and whisk until it thickens and becomes a cream.

Almond Cleansing Cream
$\frac{1}{2}$ oz. (15 g.) white wax
2 tablespoons hydrous lanolin
8 tablespoons almond oil
2 tablespoons rose water

Melt the wax and lanolin in a double boiler, beating slowly and adding the almond oil by degrees; blend in the rose water.

Avocado Cleansing Cream

½ oz. (15 g.) white wax

2 tablespoons hydrous lanolin

6 tablespoons avocado oil

5 tablespoons distilled water

Melt the wax in a double boiler, stir in the lanolin and then add the oil. Remove from the heat and slowly stir in water; stir or whisk until cool and set.

Yogurt and Lemon Cleansing Milk

1 tablespoon natural yogurt

1 teaspoon lemon juice

Simply mix together; make fresh for each use.

Cucumber Cleansing Milk

¼ cucumber

¼ pint (1·5dl.) milk

Extract or squeeze the juice from the cucumber and add to the milk; it will keep in the refrigerator for a few days.

Apple Cleansing Milk

1 apple

1 tablespoon milk

1 tablespoon fuller's earth

Put the apple through a juice extractor and combine with the milk and the fuller's earth.

Herbal Cleansing Milk

2 tablespoons elder flowers

¼ pint (1.5dl.) buttermilk

Slowly boil the flowers in the milk for half an hour, cover and leave to steep for 2 hours; strain.

FRESHENERS

Fresheners rinse away traces of oils and fats (residue from soaps and creams); they help close the pores, restore the skin's acid mantle (the pH factor), stimulate circulation and refine texture. Freshener, toner and astringent are basically the same product in graded strengths. Fresheners and toners are simple plant or herbal applications and are for balanced or dry skins. Astringents are stronger and are for oily and blemished skins. Apply by soaking cottonwool pads or gauze squares in the liquids, and wipe over the face.

Simple Skin Fresheners

Cider vinegar: Add a teaspoon to $1\frac{1}{2}$ cups water.
Potato: Rub the skin with a slice of raw potato.
Lemon: Rub with a slice of lemon, or splash with a combination of lemon juice and water.
Camphor: Put a few drops in the last rinsing water.
Cucumber: Squeeze juice of 2 cucumbers, heat to boiling point, skim away the froth, bottle and refrigerate.
Marigold: Using 6 flower heads, make an infusion, strain.
Elder flower: Using 2 cups of the flower, make an infusion, strain.
White wine: After cleansing, splash with a light white wine.

Recipes

Rose Water and Witch Hazel Toner
2 parts rose water
1 part witch hazel
Simply combine and bottle.

Orange and Lemon Toner
3 lemons
1 orange
1 cucumber
6 teaspoons rose water
$1\frac{1}{2}$ oz. (40 g.) alcohol

Extract the juice from the lemons, orange and cucumber and add the rose water and alcohol; shake well.

Lavender Toner
2 cups lavender flowers
1 oz. (30 g.) powdered orris-root
1 pint (6 dl.) vinegar

Steep the dry ingredients in the vinegar for three to four weeks; strain; dilute with an equal amount of distilled water.

ASTRINGENTS

Mild astringents are simple herbal infusions; simmer a handful of any of the following in a cup of water, allowing it to steep for a minimum of two hours: sage, bilberry leaves, parsley, fennel, camomile, yarrow.

Witch hazel has strong astringent properties and can be used on its own or as part of astringent formulas.

Simple Witch Hazel Astringent
2 parts witch hazel
3 parts rose water
Mix by shaking in a bottle.

Comfrey Astringent
$\frac{1}{2}$ teaspoon boric acid powder
1 tablespoon witch hazel
6 tablespoons comfrey infusion

Dissolve boric acid powder in the witch hazel, slowly stir in the comfrey infusion. Put immediately into a bottle, but allow to age for a minimum of a week before use.

Marigold Astringent
$\frac{1}{2}$ teaspoon alum
1 tablespoon witch hazel
6 tablespoons marigold infusion

Dissolve the alum in the witch hazel and add the marigold infusion.

Camphor Astringent
1 teaspoon spirit of camphor
4 tablespoons witch hazel
4 tablespoons rose water
4 tablespoons distilled water

Pour all the ingredients into a bottle and shake well to combine.

Almond Astringent

1 teaspoon boric acid powder

$1\frac{1}{2}$ teaspoons benzoin (friar's balsam)

1 cup rose water

2 teaspoons ground almonds

1 cup distilled water

Dissolve the boric acid powder in the benzoin, slowly add the rose water. Mix the almonds in the distilled water; combine the two liquids and shake well in a bottle.

Sage Astringent

$\frac{1}{2}$ cup dried sage

$\frac{1}{2}$ cup alcohol

$\frac{1}{4}$ teaspoon boric acid powder

3 tablespoons witch hazel

1 teaspoon glycerine

$\frac{1}{4}$ teaspoon benzoin (friar's balsam)

Steep the sage in the alcohol for a week; strain. Dissolve boric acid powder in the witch hazel and add this and all other ingredients to the sage infusion.

MOISTURIZERS

Moisturizers are preparations that form a protective film holding in the skin's moisture; they themselves do not feed moisture into the skin. Moisture is the most important aspect of skin care, as it keeps the skin supple and smooth. Dry and older skins are usually lacking in moisture. A moisturizer is applied after cleansing and the use of a freshener or astringent.

Simple Moisturizers

   Vegetable oil: A thin coating of any oil. Smooth over the face with a veil of water and blot dry.
   Cucumber: Cover the face with the juice. Blot dry.

Recipes

Basic Moisturizer

2 teaspoons white wax

1 teaspoon cocoa butter (or any vegetable margarine)

3 teaspoons coconut oil
1 teaspoon lanolin
½ teaspoon boric acid powder
4 tablespoons distilled water

Melt the wax, cocoa butter, oil and lanolin in a double boiler. Dissolve the boric acid powder in distilled water, previously warmed. Slowly beat the water into the oils until the mixture cools.

Almond Moisturizing Lotion
1 oz. (30 g.) almonds
½ pint (3 dl.) distilled water

Skin the almonds by alternately dipping in boiling and cold water and grind them to a powder. Add the distilled water drop by drop, continuing to blend until liquid is milky; strain.

Rose Water Moisturizing Lotion
5 tablespoons glycerine
3 tablespoons rose water

Pour into a bottle and shake well before each using.

Herbal Moisturizing Lotion
1 teaspoon cocoa butter
1 teaspoon lanolin
5 teaspoons almond oil
2 teaspoons herbal infusion (marigold, elder flower, comfrey, nettle, etc.)

Melt the cocoa butter, lanolin and almond oil in a double boiler; slowly add the infusion, beating constantly until cool.

Cucumber Moisturizing Cream
2 teaspoons white wax
1 teaspoon cocoa butter
3 teaspoons coconut oil
1 teaspoon lanolin
½ teaspoon boric acid powder
4 tablespoons cucumber juice
distilled water

Melt the wax, cocoa butter, oil and lanolin in a double boiler. Dissolve the boric acid powder in distilled water, previously warmed. Slowly beat in the cucumber juice.

CONDITIONERS

It is necessary to lubricate and nourish the skin with special emollients each day. This is the outward feeding of the skin that retains its smoothness and helps prevent lines and wrinkles. A thin film of conditioner is sufficient, but it should be gently massaged into the skin, using the fingertips in upward strokes over the jaw and throat areas, semi-circular movements around the eyes (very gently here) and upward arc strokes over the forehead. Leave conditioner on for a few hours or overnight. Thoroughly cleanse afterwards.

Simple Conditioners

Honey: Moisten face, massage in honey, keep on for 20 minutes, rinse away.

Honey and cream: Mix 1 teaspoon honey with 2 tablespoons light cream, beat together. Apply, leave for 20 minutes, rinse away.

Recipes

The basic recipe for a conditioning cream is one that originated in Greece many centuries ago. It was formulated by the famous doctor Galen, and to this day remains the basis for all nourishing creams. The procedure is invariably the same: first the fats are melted and the oils blended in; then any water ingredients (including herbal infusions, juices, etc.) are stirred or beaten in drop by drop; this slow process is essential and works on the same principle as adding oil to egg yolks when making mayonnaise. If it is done too quickly, the cream will be ruined.

Basic Conditioning Cream (Cold Cream)
14 oz. (400 g.) almond oil
5 oz. (150 g.) white wax
1 cup distilled water
few drops spirit vinegar

Melt the oil and wax in a double boiler; then, drop by drop, beat in the water and spirit mixture.

Simple Conditioning Cream
1 egg white
2 teaspoons honey
4 drops almond oil

Beat the egg white and add it to the honey, stir in the oil; refrigerate – it only lasts a few days.

Sesame Oil Cream
½ oz. (15 g.) white wax
1 oz. (30 g.) lanolin
1 oz. (30 g.) spermaceti
5 oz. (150 g.) sesame oil
2½ oz. (75 g.) rose water
Melt all the fats and oil in a double boiler and slowly add the rose water.

Orange Blossom Cream
½ oz. (15 g.) white wax
2 oz. (60 g.) almond oil
½ oz. (15 g.) spermaceti
1 oz. (30 g.) orange blossom infusion
Melt oils and fats together in a double boiler and slowly add the orange blossom infusion.

Lily and Marshmallow Cream
1 tablespoon marshmallow root infusion
½ pint (3dl.) distilled water
1 tablespoon lily bulb powder
1 tablespoon honey
1 teaspoon rose water
1 oz. (30 g.) lanolin
The marshmallow infusion is made by steeping the finely chopped root in cold water for a few hours; the liquid becomes gelatinous – strain before use. Simmer this together with the distilled water and lily bulb powder for half an hour. Strain. Add the honey and rose water and blend well. Melt the lanolin in a double boiler and slowly add the above mixture.

Comfrey Cream
2 tablespoons lanolin
3 tablespoons white wax
4 tablespoons almond oil
¼ teaspoon boric acid powder
1 tablespoon distilled water
1 tablespoon strong comfrey infusion

Melt the lanolin and wax in a double boiler and add the oil; dissolve the boric acid powder in the distilled water and add slowly to the melted fats; finally slowly beat in the comfrey infusion.

Simple Marigold Cream
1 large jar Vaseline
6 marigold heads

Melt the Vaseline in a double boiler, break up the flower heads, drop into the liquid and simmer for two hours – very gently. Strain before pouring into jars.

Strawberry Conditioning Cream
2 teaspoons lanolin
2 teaspoons powdered oatmeal
½ cup fresh or frozen strawberry juice

Melt the lanolin in a double boiler, add the oatmeal and when mixture is smooth stir in the strawberry juice, beating all the time as the drops are added.

EXFOLIATORS

Otherwise known as thinners or peelers, exfoliators help remove the dead surface cells. If these are not taken away, the skin becomes flaky or rough, often mottled in appearance. In addition, the dead cells clog up the pores and prevent normal skin activity.

Exfoliators are abrasive; some astringents (see page 162) act as mild thinners and are fine for young skins. Older skins require something tougher. Exfoliate once a week, after cleansing; once the treatment is finished, rinse the skin, then moisturize it.

Vegetable oil: Rub the face with any vegetable oil, then dab on a film of warm water and a layer of apple cider vinegar. Rub in this mixture with circular movements; it will flake and peel off, taking the dead cells with it.

Salt: Sprinkle ordinary salt on a wet facecloth and rub onto the face, but not too hard; rinse away. Not for use on delicate skin.

Papaya mint tea: Pour 2 cups of boiling water on 2 papaya mint tea bags and leave to steep for a few minutes; soak a facecloth in the tea; wring out; apply to the face holding cloth against the skin. The tea must be hot to be effective; keep heating and renewing cloth. Continue applications for 15 minutes.

FACIALS

Facials cleanse, stimulate and nourish the skin; they also increase circulation, bringing nutrients and oxygen to the surface. They often contain ingredients that act as purifiers, drawing out dirt, toxins and grease. Facials are usually in mask form, though sometimes a steam procedure is used. The face has to be thoroughly cleansed with a final clear water rinse before commencing any facial treatment.

Steam Facials

Herbal steam facials encourage the pores to push out dirt and impurities, while at the same time they help to heal blemishes. Pour boiling water over the herbs in a bowl; make a towel into a head tent and steam the face over the bowl for 10 minutes. Blot dry, freshen and moisturize. Traditionally the following herbs have been used in steam facials, either singly or combined. (An infusion of any of the following can also be added to the solid masks with the same effects.)

For cleansing, soothing: camomile, lady's mantle, nettle, rosemary, thyme, marigold.
For tightening: peppermint, elder flower, benzoin, gum arabic.
For drying: yarrow.
For healing: leek, comfrey, fennel.

Solid Facials

Fruits, vegetables and herbs can be used alone, mixed or combined with a thickener (a substance that binds the ingredients together giving the facial a firm professional quality).

Basically, a fruit or vegetable is mashed, an infusion is made of a herb. If the mixture is too runny, it is given substance by adding one of the following: oatmeal, fuller's earth, clay, kaolin, honey and mashed banana – all neutral binders; whipped egg white or yogurt – these help oily skin conditions; whipped egg yolk or honey – these help dry skin.

To make a slightly acid mantle, add a few drops of apple cider vinegar or fresh lemon juice.

If the facial skin is dry or rough, add about a tablespoon of oil – almond, avocado, olive, safflower or wheatgerm.

To help retain moisture, use honey or glycerine, which attract water from the under layers of the skin; or add the contents of a vitamin E capsule (100 international units) to the facial.

It is not difficult to gauge the right consistency. A mask needs to be just thick enough to smooth on the face without running off; start by adding the binder slowly to avoid making the formula too stiff. A mask is applied to a clean, rinsed face and should be kept on for 20 minutes. Some harden and dry, tightening the skin at the same time – but this depends on the binding material. The eye area should be left free and covered with milk-soaked pads. Lie down the entire time, with the head a little lower than the body if possible. Masks rinse off easily with warm water.

Simple Facials

Strawberry: Freshly mashed and applied, this softens and lightens the skin and helps balance the pH factor; mix with oatmeal if too sloppy.

Pineapple: Enzymatic action helps clear away dead-cell debris. Soak gauze pads in the juice and leave on the face for the usual 20 minutes.

Apricot: Mash fresh ones to a pulp – or soak dried ones overnight – cook until soft, then mash. Add a binder if necessary.

Grape: Use seedless green grapes, mashed to a pulp. For dry skin add honey or a beaten egg yolk; for oily skin add a whisked egg white.

Avocado: Mash, and mix with honey and lemon juice.

Tomato: Mash and combine with oatmeal.

Cucumber: Mash, and add binder if desired.

Cabbage: Extract juice from very green leaves and heat slightly; soak gauze pads in the juice to apply.

Egg white: Whisk until stiff and brush on; $\frac{1}{4}$ teaspoon of cider vinegar may be added to balance the acid mantle of the skin. Alternatively, whisk the egg white with a tablespoon of skimmed milk.

Egg yolk: Beat, and combine with a tablespoon of honey and a teaspoon of any vegetable oil.

Honey: 2 tablespoons honey and $\frac{1}{2}$ teaspoon of lemon juice or cider vinegar.

Brewer's yeast: 1 teaspoon powdered yeast and about 2 teaspoons warm water; adjust the consistency so that it will spread like a paste.

Recipes for Facials

Apricot Facial
6 dried apricots
2 cups cold milk
1 teaspoon avocado or almond oil
1 teaspoon honey
3 drops apple cider vinegar

Soak the apricots in milk overnight, remove from the liquid and mash well. Add the oil, honey and cider vinegar; pat on to the face.

Apple Facial
1 apple
$\frac{1}{2}$ teaspoon cream
1 tablespoon honey
1 tablespoon ground oatmeal

Mash the apple with the cream, add the honey and oatmeal.

Oatmeal Facial
2 tablespoons unprocessed oatmeal
$\frac{1}{2}$ cup milk
2 teaspoons elder flower water

Cook the oatmeal and milk as though it were porridge until soft. Remove from the heat, add the elder flower water and beat together. When it is just warm spread it over the face.

Mayonnaise Facial
1 cup olive oil
1 egg
$\frac{1}{2}$ teaspoon sea-salt
2 tablespoons lemon juice

Blend half a cup of the oil with the remaining ingredients; whip until thick and pour in the rest of the oil very slowly. Keep refrigerated.

Honey Facial
1 egg yolk
1 teaspoon olive oil
1 tablespoon honey

Beat the egg yolk into the oil, then blend in the honey.

Honey and Oatmeal Facial

1 oz. (30 g.) honey

1 teaspoon lemon juice

2 unbeaten egg whites

½ teaspoon almond oil

2 tablespoons powdered oatmeal

Mix everything together except the oatmeal. When smooth slowly add sufficient oatmeal to make a moist, but not sloppy, paste.

Wheatgerm Facial

1 egg yolk

½ teaspoon wheatgerm

¾ cup of almond oil

1 teaspoon distilled water

Beat the first three ingredients together, add the water and beat again. Brush on the face.

Cucumber Facial

1 cucumber

¼ teaspoon lemon juice

1 teaspoon witch hazel

1 teaspoon alcohol

1 egg white, whipped

Peel the cucumber and extract the juice; add the lemon juice, witch hazel and alcohol. Stir well; then blend in the whipped egg.

DRY SKIN

Dry skin requires constant lubrication to prevent flaking and premature ageing. One of the easiest ways to counteract it is to put oil in the daily bath (see Bathing, page 183 for special bath oil formulas). A few drops of any vegetable oil suffices and it doesn't matter if it is not an oil that disperses in water, as floating oil will cling to the skin and work just as well. Alternatively, an oil-based shampoo can be added to the bath – it provides bubbles as well. Use a creamy body lotion after bathing.

CLEANSING: Almond oil is good for dry skin, otherwise any of the cream cleansers (see page 159). Particularly recommended is the following, with a cocoa butter base.

Dry Skin Cleanser
1 tablespoon cocoa butter
1 tablespoon anhydrous lanolin
3 tablespoons almond oil

Melt everything in a double boiler, or a glass bowl placed in boiling water; it is important to be sure that all the fats are well dissolved before cooling.

FRESHENING: Any of the fresheners given on page 161. Never use an astringent – it is too strong.

CONDITIONING: Daily with one of the rich emollients listed on pages 165–7.

FACIALS: Refer to the recipes for facials (page 169) – all those containing oil, honey or egg yolk can be used. Simple facials are made more beneficial by adding a teaspoon of a lubricating oil – avocado, wheatgerm, sesame or olive; it is also advantageous to add a few drops of apple cider vinegar. The best binders are honey, egg yolk or mashed banana. Best fruits and vegetables are avocado, artichoke heart, strawberry, apricot, tomato, cucumber and papaya.

OILY SKIN

Oily skin is invariably blemished; it may have pimples, even acne (special remedies for these conditions, see pages 175–6). Skin care here is aimed at preventing the pores from becoming clogged with oil and dirt and thus susceptible to infection.

CLEANSING: Remove make-up with skimmed milk, it is easiest to make it from the powder – 2 teaspoons per cup of warm water. Oatmeal moistened with lemon juice is good for cleaning out the pores. Otherwise a mild alkaline soap works equally well.

FRESHENING: Astringents are usually necessary for oily skins (see page 162). Simple remedies are

    the juice of half a lemon in a cup of water
    rub over with a slice of raw potato
    a teaspoon of apple cider vinegar in a cup of water
    cucumber, lettuce, cabbage or carrot juice
    an infusion of parsley

CONDITIONING: Oily skins rarely require additional lubrication unless there are isolated dry areas. Here is a fat-free formula for use as a refining cream.

Oily Skin Cream
1 teaspoon natural pectin powder
1 oz. (30 g.) alcohol
½ oz. (15 g.) glycerine
1½ oz. (45 g.) rose water

Mix the pectin powder with a little of the alcohol and slowly add the glycerine, then the rest of the alcohol and lastly the rose water. Bring the mixture to the boil and keep bubbling for 3 minutes; cool.

FACIALS: A very important part of oily skin care, as they can dry and purify the skin. All facial formulas are beneficial (see page 169) but binding agents when used should be yogurt, buttermilk, egg white, fuller's earth or kaolin. Avoid those containing honey and egg yolk. The addition of a teaspoon of lemon juice is valuable because of its astringent quality, and so is apple cider vinegar (½ teaspoon). Two recipes are specially useful:

Cucumber Facial
½ cup peeled and chopped cucumber
2 teaspoons powdered milk
1 egg white

Mash the cucumber and add powdered milk and finally the egg white; it is more efficient to mix the ingredients in a blender.

Brewer's Yeast Facial
3 tablespoons of yogurt
2 tablespoons brewer's yeast

Add the yogurt slowly to the brewer's yeast powder, making quite a sloppy mixture; brush on to the face.

WRINKLES

Wrinkles cannot be removed but they can be softened and their appearance delayed. Oil is a great help, taken in the diet or gently patted on to the face – areas around the eyes and the mouth are the first to register lines. Use almond or turtle oil.

Wrinkle lotion: Bathe with an infusion of camomile, lemon balm or chervil.

Apricot Wrinkle Cream
2 tablespoons lanolin
1 tablespoon apricot oil
1 teaspoon lemon juice
3 drops benzoin
Melt lanolin in a glass bowl in a pan of simmering water; stir in the apricot oil and lemon juice; blend very well and finally add the benzoin; beat again.

Wrinkle facial: Beat the white of an egg together with 3 drops of lemon juice; brush on the face and allow to dry thoroughly before rinsing off.

MATURE SKIN

Apart from becoming lined and wrinkled (see immediately above for aids) it can be loose and flabby, particularly if there has been any quick and considerable weight loss.

Skin Firming Lotion
1 tablespoon fresh cucumber juice
3 tablespoons rose water or elder flower water
1 teaspoon benzoin
Mix all ingredients together and strain; apply twice a day.

Skin Tightening Mask
1 egg white
1 tablespoon powdered milk
½ teaspoon honey
Beat together until thoroughly blended, brush on the face and allow to dry for 20 minutes. Rinse away. This will tighten skin but only for a few hours.

Neck and Throat Firming Mask
1 egg white
1 teaspoon honey
2 teaspoons milk
1 teaspoon spirit of camphor

Mix well, brush on the throat and leave until dry. Rinse away; be sure to moisturize well afterwards.

BLEMISHED SKIN

Break-outs on the skin, whether mild clusters of spots that are more like a rash, pimples or the more serious acne, can be considerably helped by persevering with natural aids. Firstly, suggestions for minor blemishes:

Carrot facial: Finely grate 3 medium-size carrots. Apply to the skin; leave on for 20 minutes, rinse off.

Parsley lotion: Steep a handful of parsley in a cup of boiling water for about 30 minutes. Strain, and apply in compress form to the face for 10 to 15 minutes a day until troubled skin is cleared.

Egg white: One beaten egg white plus 2 drops spirit of camphor. Dab on pimples, leave on for 20 minutes to dry and wash off. Or combine 1 egg white with 1 tablespoon of mashed cucumber and apply as a facial.

Cucumber Facial for Pimples
1 cucumber
$\frac{1}{2}$ teaspoon lemon juice
1 tablespoon vodka (or alcohol)
8 drops peppermint extract
3 drops spirit of camphor

Peel and slice cucumber, mash to a pulp and add the remaining ingredients. Pat on the face and leave for just 10 minutes – with repeated use blemishes should dry up.

Pimple Clearing Cream
2 sliced apples
2 tablespoons chopped fennel
2 tablespoons chopped celery
$\frac{1}{4}$ oz. (7 g.) barley meal
2 pints (1 l.) rose water
3 egg whites
1 teaspoon lanolin

In a double boiler, simmer the apples, fennel, celery and barley meal in the rose water; when mushy add beaten egg white and lanolin. Strain and beat until smooth. Keep in the refrigerator.

Basic Pimple Cream
1 tablespoon castor oil
1 tablespoon glycerine
1 tablespoon lanolin

Melt all ingredients together in a glass bowl placed in simmering water; cool.

BLACKHEADS

Almond meal cleanser: 1 cup almond meal and about $\frac{1}{2}$ cup water; combine to make a foamy consistency; work over the face using a fine-bristled brush to get into the pores, but do not scrub too hard. Rinse off.

Bicarbonate of soda compresses: Dissolve 1 teaspoon of bicarbonate of soda in a cup of hot water. Soak gauze or cotton pads in the liquid and apply to the blackhead ruptures as hot as possible to open clogged pores.

Parsley lotion: Soak a bunch of parsley overnight, preferably in a non-gaseous mineral water. Strain; dip cottonwool balls in the liquid and apply to the afflicted areas. This is also good as a general cleanser for oily skin.

White wine wash: A light Sauterne or Rhine wine is considered the best. Combine 1 cup with the juice of a lemon and wash the blackhead surfaces with it. The wine can also be used to moisten a dish of oatmeal, making a paste that can be rubbed into the skin.

Iodine lotion: Dissolve 1 tablespoon Epsom salts in a cup of boiling water, add 3 drops iodine; apply hot.

ACNE

Papaya mint tea compresses: Steep 1 papaya mint tea bag in a teacup of hot water until a strong brew is obtained; reheat to boiling point. Soak gauze or cottonwool pads in the tea and pat on the affected areas as hot as the skin can bear.

Burdock steam facial: Simmer 2 handfuls of dried burdock leaves in 2 cups of water for 5 minutes and strain. Return to the pot for reheating when necessary. Dip a terry facecloth or small towel into the warm liquid and hold against the face. Repeat for 15 minutes keeping the infusion at a temperature high enough for steaming.

Calcium helps acne; sunflower seeds are a good source and so are supplements of bonemeal.

FRECKLES

Freckles usually appear with age or because of over-exposure to the sun, though some people are simply born with them as a genetic heritage. There are ways to lessen or lighten them, though they can rarely be removed.

Yogurt: Daily applications of natural yogurt.

Cranberry: Crush fresh cranberries and rub into the skin.

Watercress: Combine the juice of a bunch of watercress with a teaspoon of honey; apply as a mask.

Castor oil: Simply rub in the crude oil.

Simple Freckle Cream

¼ cup of sour milk (or buttermilk)

½ teaspoon grated horse-radish

1 tablespoon powdered oatmeal

Mix all the ingredients together to a paste and apply to the freckled areas, but keep clear of the eyes; leave on for 30 minutes.

Elder Flower Freckle Cream

1 teaspoon alum

1 tablespoon lemon juice

2 tablespoons elder flower water

Mix all the ingredients together; this paste is quite runny, so brush it on freckled areas; leave for 30 minutes.

WARTS

Dandelion: The white sap from the stalk can be used to dry out warts; several applications are necessary.

Greater celandine: The orange-coloured juice that comes from the stalk will discolour and dry out warts; again several applications are needed.

SUNTANNING

Coconut oil: Use it as it is – it will harden when cool, but melts very quickly in the sun.

Olive oil: Combine with an equal quantity of apple cider vinegar.

Sesame seeds: Grind a handful of seeds, add enough water to cover and a bit extra; beat until a milky lotion emerges.

Sesame oil is actually about the best natural protector there is, and it is the basis of many protective formulas. The following preparations protect in varying degrees, depending upon the type of skin you have. As with all rules on sunbathing, they should be used sensibly and exposure to the sun should be gradual and never excessive.

Sesame Tanning Lotion
$\frac{1}{4}$ cup lanolin
$\frac{1}{4}$ cup sesame oil
$\frac{3}{4}$ cup distilled water

In a double boiler, melt the lanolin; take off the heat and blend with sesame oil and water. Keep in the refrigerator.

Citrus Tanning Oil
$\frac{1}{2}$ cup sesame oil
8 drops of citronella

Put in a bottle and shake well; this also gives protection against insect bites.

Tea Tanning Lotion
1 tablespoon lanolin
4 tablespoons sesame oil
4 tablespoons strong cold Indian tea

Melt the lanolin and the oil in a double boiler. Remove from the heat and stir in the cold tea.

Cocoa Butter Lotion
$\frac{1}{4}$ cup cocoa butter
$\frac{1}{4}$ cup almond oil
2 drops verbena oil

First melt the cocoa butter together with the almond oil in a double boiler, then remove from heat and stir in the verbena drops.

Iodine Bronzing Lotion
1 cup sesame oil
10 drops iodine
juice of a lemon

Blend all ingredients together and shake well before using.

Sun Protection Lotion
1 peeled cucumber
$\frac{1}{2}$ teaspoon glycerine
$\frac{1}{2}$ teaspoon rose water

Extract the juice from the cucumber and mix with the glycerine and rose water; refrigerate.

SUNBURN

To ease sunburn, if the skin is red and painful, try these antidotes:

equal parts of baking soda and water, patted on and left for half an hour

a strong infusion of ordinary cold tea or sage tea

a pulp of mashed strawberries or cucumber, left on for half an hour

take a bath to which has been added a cup of bicarbonate of soda

splash burned areas with a diluted solution of cider vinegar and water

mix $\frac{1}{4}$ cup of buttermilk (or yogurt) with 2 tablespoons rose water; splash over the skin

break up a cake of yeast, mash into $\frac{1}{2}$ cup of cider vinegar and blend well – cools the skin

beat the white of an egg with 1 teaspoon of castor oil and smooth over skin as a lotion.

Anti-Sunburn Cream
1 egg white
1 teaspoon honey
$\frac{1}{2}$ teaspoon witch hazel

Beat the egg white, blend in honey and then the witch hazel; smooth over sunburn. This must be kept in the refrigerator.

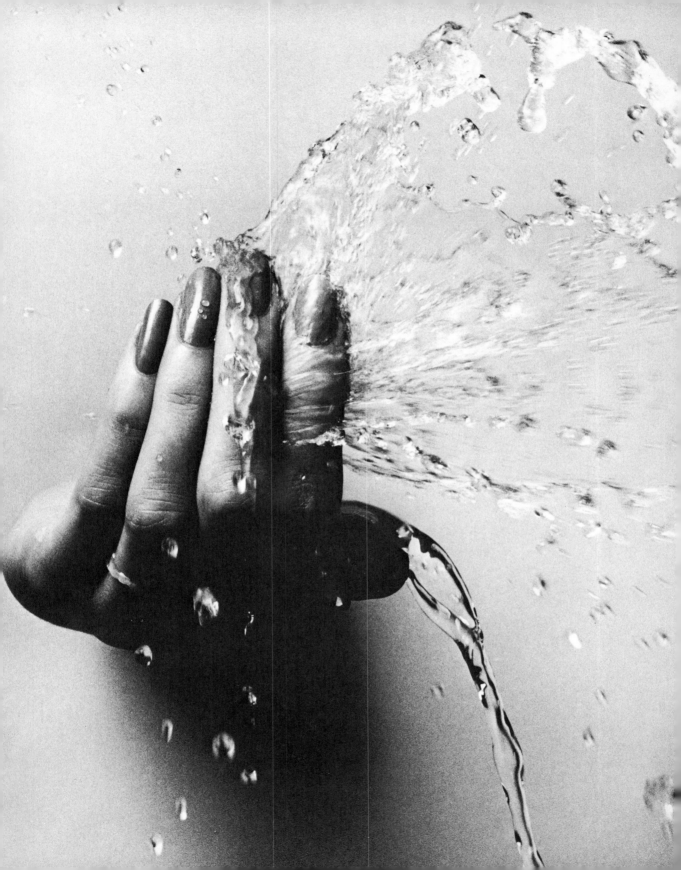

2

BATHING

Herbs, oils and fragrances can transform bathing into a therapeutic treatment. It can relax or stimulate; at the same time it can soften, lubricate, tone and scent the skin.

Herbs may be used in the bath alone or in combination. Dried or fresh herbs can be put in a cheesecloth bag which hangs over the tap or is immersed in the bath. Or they can be made into an infusion like a tea – a pint (6 dl.) of boiling water to 2 tablespoons of leaves or flowers. Do not boil the herbs; pour boiling water over them and steep for a minimum of 15 minutes. Use mint, lavender and rosemary for energy and revitalizing the body and mind, cedar and pine for relaxation and meditation, jasmine and camomile for soothing the nerves, rose, elder flower and marigold for calming, comfrey for healing and carnation for overall well-being.

Mint Bath – to refresh
1 cup pine needles
1 cup peppermint leaves
2 drops oil of rosemary
Mix dry ingredients; add oil and stir well. Put into cheesecloth bags.

Lemon Bath – to cool
1 cup lemon verbena
1 cup lemon balm
3 drops oil of lemon
Mix first three ingredients, add oil; put into cheesecloth bags.

Spicy Bath – to warm
1 cup elder flowers
1 cup blackberry leaves
1 cup rose geranium leaves
2 drops rose geranium oil

Mix all the ingredients and add the oil; put into cheesecloth bags.

Lavender Mix Bath – to revive
1 cup dried lavender flowers
$\frac{1}{2}$ cup mint leaves
$\frac{1}{2}$ cup rosemary
$\frac{1}{4}$ cup powdered comfrey root

Put all ingredients into a fine muslin bag; pour on boiling water and steep for 3 minutes. Pour liquid into bath.

Bay Leaf Bath – for strained muscles
$\frac{1}{2}$ cup bay leaves
2 cups water

Simmer for 5 minutes, then steep for 15. Strain and pour directly into the bath.

Coconut Oil Bath – to soften
8 oz. (225 g.) coconut oil
2 cups elder flowers
6 drops tincture of benzoin

Melt the coconut oil in the top of a double boiler, transfer to a glass or earthenware pot, add the elder flowers and simmer for 2 hours. Strain, add the benzoin and bottle.

Grain Bath – for rough skin
$\frac{1}{2}$ cup barley
$\frac{1}{2}$ cup rice
$\frac{1}{2}$ cup bran
3 quarts (3.4 l.) of water

Soak the grains first for about an hour, then simmer the mixture for an hour. Strain and use about 2 cups per bath.

Bicarbonate of Soda Bath – to calm or to stop itching
3 cups bicarbonate of soda
1 drop oil of rosemary
1 drop oil of lavender

Simply put the bicarbonate of soda in a jar; add the oils and allow to stand a week before use, shaking the mixture every so often. If you prefer a more heady oriental fragrance, substitute 2 drops of ylang-ylang for the rosemary and lavender. Use $1\frac{1}{2}$ cups to a bath – its alkaline action soothes the skin and helps banish perspiration odours.

Cider Vinegar Bath – a skin aid   1 cup of cider vinegar added to the bath restores the acid mantle of the skin; the odour of vinegar does not stay.

Seaweed Bath – to tone skin   Fill a muslin bag with fresh or dried seaweed and allow it to soak in a warm bath for 10 minutes before bathing.

Milk and Honey Bath – to nourish skin
$1\frac{3}{4}$ oz. (55 g.) bicarbonate of soda
4 oz. (120 g.) salt
3 pints (1·8 l.) milk
1 lb. (450 g.) honey

Dissolve soda and salt in a pint (6 dl.) of lukewarm water. Make 3 pints (1·8 l.) of milk from dried milk following the proportions indicated on the package; warm it and add the honey. First put the soda-and-salt mixture in a warm bath, then stir in the milk and honey.

Milk Bath – to nourish   1 cup of powdered skimmed milk in a bath of warm water – today's economical version of the traditional milk bath.

Oatmeal Bath – to nourish   1 lb. (450 g.) of oatmeal, stirred into the bath or enclosed in a muslin bag.

BATH OILS

The simplest way to keep the skin well lubricated is to add oil to the bath. It has to be a vegetable oil, and the only one that makes a good dispersing agent (meaning that drops of oil will mix with the water) is specially treated castor oil, sometimes known as turkey red oil. All other oils will float on top of the water and will only get on to your skin as you get out of the bath.

Simple Aromatic Oil
¾ cup treated castor oil
¼ cup any aromatic oil – pleasing fragrances are rose, jasmine, lavender, mint, pine, lemon flower, orange blossom

Mix oils together and use 1 – 2 teaspoons per bath.

Verbena Bath Oil
¾ cup treated castor oil
½ cup alcohol (or vodka)
1 tablespoon lemon verbena

Shake all together in a bottle and use a tablespoon in the bath.

Almond Bath Oil
1 cup almond oil
1 tablespoon liquid castile shampoo
1 teaspoon rose geranium oil

Shake well, and always shake before use – about a tablespoon per bath.

Lavender Soothing Oil
2 tablespoons sesame oil
3 drops oil of lavender
2 tablespoons gum arabic (powdered)
1 cup water

Shake the oils together. Put the gum arabic in a separate bowl and add the combined oils drop by drop. Make a smooth paste and then slowly add the water, finally beating the mixture until the whole cup has been added. Use 2 teaspoonfuls in a bath (preferably not until 24 hours after making), and store in the refrigerator if possible. It is particularly silky and soothing.

Bubble Bath Oil
½ cup shredded castile soap
1½ cups hot water
2 teaspoons witch hazel
1½ tablespoons glycerine
3 drops of either rose, rose geranium or lavender oil

Melt the soap in the hot water. In another bowl combine the witch hazel, glycerine and fragrant oil and then add to the soapy mixture. Use about 2 tablespoons per bath.

Musky Bubble Bath
2 cups mild soap flakes
3 drops lavender oil
3 drops bergamot oil
3 drops tincture of musk

Combine all ingredients and allow to stand for a week before use; 2 tablespoons per bath.

DEODORANTS

Natural produce can help counteract odour, but cannot control wetness. It is the chlorophyll in green vegetables that does the job, so drink the juices and eat the vegetables rich in this substance: parsley, watercress, green cabbage, the outer dark leaves of lettuce, beet tops, spinach.

Lettuce: Break up and mash the green leaves; brush the resultant green liquid under the arms.

Parsley: Use in the same way as lettuce.

Chrysanthemum: The leaves are very good for controlling odour; make an infusion, bottle and use regularly.

Sage: Use an infusion under the arms or in the bath.

Lovage: Lovage in a hot bath acts as a deodorant and purifier; put the shredded leaves in a muslin bag.

Apple cider vinegar: Dilute with 2 parts distilled water to neutralize odour; the aroma of vinegar disappears in about 15 minutes. It is better to apply it with cottonwool pads, as fingers often retain the smell.

Lavender oil: Dilute for underarm use: mix together 3 drops lavender oil, 1 tablespoon sugar and 1 pint (6 dl.) distilled water; leave for 2 weeks. Always shake before use.

VAGINAL DOUCHES

Natural douches are the best cleansers, but constant douching is undesirable as it can destroy beneficial bacteria and upset the natural balance.

Apple cider vinegar or white vinegar: Use ½ cup to 6 cups of water.
Rosemary: Use a mild infusion, well strained; ½ cup to 5 cups of water.
Rose geranium leaves: An infusion of 1 cup to 4 cups of water, strained.
Lightly salted warm water: This is also efficient.

TALCUM POWDER

One basic recipe suffices; any perfume you choose can be added to it in the
form of essential oil.

Basic Powder
5 oz. (150 g.) rice flour
5 oz. (150 g.) talcum of precipitated chalk
6 teaspoons powdered orris-root
3 teaspoons boric acid powder
1 teaspoon any essential oil

Mix together the rice flour, chalk and orris-root, add the boric acid powder
and mix well. Add any essential oil, a single one or a combination of several,
but in all not more than a teaspoon. Stir well until oils are completely
absorbed within the powders. Sift two or three times.

SOAP

The idea of making soap at home sounds formidable, but it is easier than
many normal cooking procedures. It is, however, absolutely necessary to
measure quantities exactly and to control temperatures. The saponification
process depends upon a chemical interaction, so mass and heat regulation is
important.

The fundamentals are simple. All soap is made the same way with the
optional additions of a lubricating substance, a herbal infusion, vegetable
and fruit pulps, perfume and colour. The two main ingredients are caustic
soda (which is mixed with water) and fat – which can be lard, vegetable
margarine, tallow or oil. The fat is heated in a large cauldron until it reaches
a certain temperature, usually between 90° and 110° F (32° and 43° C). In
another container, the caustic soda (sometimes known as lye) is added to
water, and its temperature adjusted to be a little cooler than that of the fat.
The two are then stirred together until they interact and the mixture

thickens like custard. This can take from 20 to 30 minutes. It is then poured into moulds to harden and mature.

Utensils are also very important. Because caustic soda can badly damage aluminium, tin or foil, always use stainless steel or enamel pots for heating the fats, and glass containers for mixing the caustic soda. Be sure there are no chips or cracks in the enamel, nor any flaws in the glassware. Always use wooden spoons for mixing and stirring.

Caustic soda is not pleasant to work with and it should be treated with caution. Wear plastic gloves. If even a speck gets on your skin, wash immediately with lots of water – preferably water mixed with vinegar – otherwise you may get a painful burn. Also, when the caustic soda is added to the water, the fumes and smell are terrible – try not to breathe them in.

Moulds can be cardboard or plastic containers; actually various sizes of small cardboard boxes are the best for they hold the soap in its liquid state and prevent it from cooling too quickly. They have to be lined with a damp cloth or two layers of wet brown paper. This ensures that the soap can be lifted out easily without ruining its shape – the cloth and paper simply peel off. It is also advisable to put the boxes on newspaper while the soap is solidifying, as the caustic soda may sometimes seep through. Patterned objects can be put on the bottom of the mould for decoration – even a piece of heavily embossed brocade will provide an adequate impression. But take care not to use anything that will be damaged by the caustic soda.

Basic Soap Recipe (about 4 bars of soap)
4 cups lard or margarine
2 cups water (distilled or tap)
5 tablespoons caustic soda (crystals or flakes)

First prepare the caustic soda solution – pour the water into a glass bowl or a large jar and stir in the caustic soda until it dissolves. Take care – great heat is generated, and a fair amount of bubbling and spluttering. It will heat up immediately to about 200°F (93°C). It must, however, cool down to between 85° and 90°F (29° and 32°C) before it can be combined with the fats.

Now prepare the fat, by bringing the lard or margarine to melting point in an enamelled or stainless-steel pot. Remove from the heat and cool to a temperature of 90°F (32°C).

The caustic soda should be a few degrees cooler than the melted fat. With the pot of fat off the burner, slowly add the caustic soda. It is extremely important always to add the caustic soda solution to the fat; never the reverse. Stir with a wooden spoon. The fat will at first turn pink, then it will begin to lighten and finally it will become white.

Stir slowly and evenly. It takes 20 to 30 minutes, but it does not have to be stirred constantly – you can take a minute's break every now and then.

When the mixture has the consistency of a sauce, neither runny nor too thick, pour it into the prepared moulds, cover with cardboard or a towel, wrap in another towel to prevent cooling too fast and leave in a warm dry place to set. This should take 24 hours, but sometimes needs a little longer. Remove from the mould, peel off the paper or cloths, cut with a taut piece of wire, wrap in greaseproof paper and leave for at least 2 weeks.

If the soap mixture does not thicken, it could be because it is too warm, so cool it by standing in cold water for a while, stirring continually. If it still does not thicken, try heating again to $100°-110°$ F $(38°-43°$ C) and repeating the stirring process.

Sometimes the soap curdles, and nothing can be done about it – except throw it away. This happens when the temperatures are wrong, the quantities unbalanced or the fat rancid.

The optional additions – perfume, colour and nutrients – may be added just before pouring into the moulds, stirring for a few minutes to make sure of even distribution and texture.

Scent: This has to be added carefully; just a couple of drops for the quantities detailed above. Recommended are lavender, bergamot, rose geranium, verbena and patchouli; if desired, two fragrant oils can be combined (a drop of each) but never more.

Colour: Something else that has to be added with caution. Food colourings can be used, but in very small amounts, otherwise the colour can transfer itself to the skin, albeit temporarily. It is preferable to use natural colourants.

Greens – spinach gives various hues of green depending on the strength of the infusion. Bruise the dark leaves, just cover with water and simmer until the liquid is coloured; continue until the volume is reduced by half in order to obtain a strong tone. Refrigerate if not used immediately.

Yellow to orange – saffron provides this range; it is expensive, but only a pinch is needed. Put in a glass jar, pour over it $\frac{1}{2}$ cup boiling water; leave to stand for several days, shaking every so often; strain before using.

Pink to red – from the alkanet root (obtainable from a herbalist); put $\frac{1}{2}$ oz. (15 g.) in a glass bottle, add $\frac{1}{2}$ pint (3 dl.) vodka; allow to steep for a week, shaking several times a day; strain. Again the range from pale pink to a deep red must be judged by eye and can be controlled by adding the colouring drop by drop.

Beige to brown – burnt sugar will provide this range. Put $\frac{1}{2}$ oz. (15 g.) sugar in a heavy frying pan and heat slowly until it turns dark brown, almost black; remove from the heat and cover with a cup of water; steep for 10 minutes but stir all the time; strain.

Nutrients: 2 tablespoons of any of the following will add texture as well as nourishment – mashed avocado, strawberry, cucumber, oatmeal (soaked first) or ground almonds.

Honey Soap
$6\frac{1}{2}$ oz. (180 g.) caustic soda
20 oz. (570 g.) water
45 oz. (1·25 kg.) fat – lard or tallow
3 oz. (85 g.) coconut oil
2 oz. (55 g.) honey
2 drops essential oil (your choice)
burnt sugar colouring

Follow the basic procedure; caustic soda and water should be at 100°F (38°C), the fats at 110°F (43°C). Add honey, colouring (to the degree desired) and fragrance just before pouring into moulds; stir well first.

Glycerine Soap
$6\frac{1}{2}$ oz. (180 g.) caustic soda
20 oz. (570 g.) water
45 oz. (1·25 kg.) fat – lard or tallow
3 oz (85 g.) glycerine
dark pink colouring (see above)
3 drops oil of rose geranium

Follow the basic procedure; caustic soda and water should be at 98°F (37°C), fats at 110°F (43°C). Add the glycerine as the soap begins to thicken slightly, then the colour and finally the oil of rose geranium.

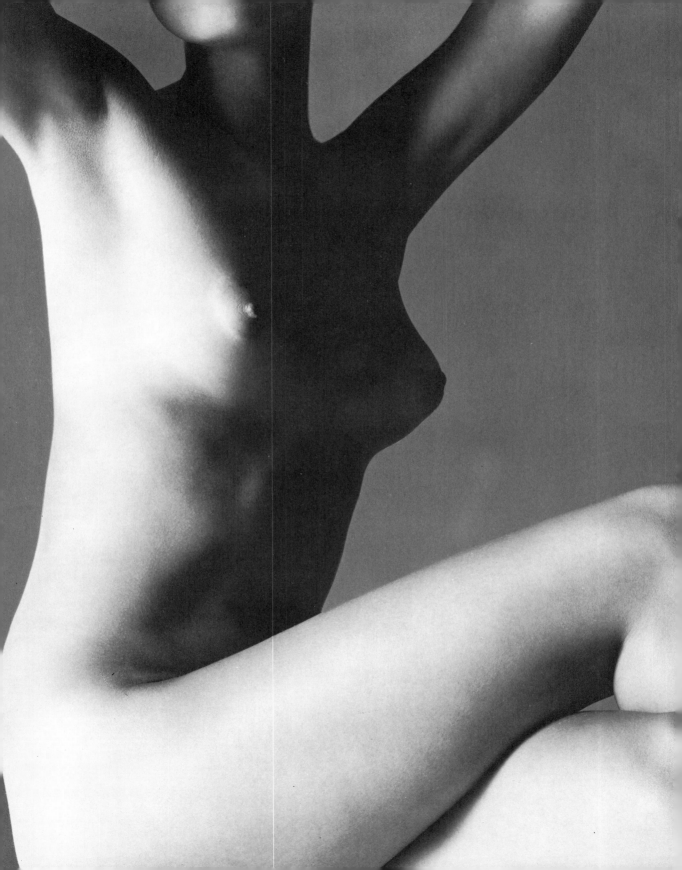

3

BODY

The general condition of the body depends on the healthful elements that go into it, the régimes that are followed, the prevention methods that are taken, etc. However, many visible and external problems can also be helped by using treatments of natural origin.

CELLULITE

This dimpled, stubborn fat which mainly accumulates on the thighs, buttocks, hips and upper arms is due to a combination of excess fat and excess water retention. Natural ways to help it involve diet, special vegetable juices and tisanes, compresses to help ease out the water and a herbal friction lotion to aid in the tightening of the skin surface.

Cellulite Diet

Morning: on waking, immediately drink a glass of hot water with the juice of $\frac{1}{2}$ lemon.

Breakfast: (to be taken 20 minutes after the lemon drink) mixed vegetable juices, $\frac{1}{2}$ pint (3 dl.) in all – $\frac{1}{3}$ each of cucumber, beet (boiled) and carrot juice; a fresh fruit salad, but no banana.

Lunch: $\frac{1}{2}$ pint (3 dl.) of the same juice mix; fresh green salad, dressed with lemon juice, olive oil, herbs for flavouring and a little sea-salt.

Dinner: 1 sliced ripe tomato topped with lemon juice and a drop of oil, touch of sea-salt, basil or marjoram for flavouring; 2 steamed non-starch vegetables – spring beans, cabbage, carrots, zucchini or celery – topped with a smudge of butter; 2 slices broiled liver or lean meat.

Bedtime: a glass of celery juice (to induce sound sleep).

Drinks: herbal tea (equal parts of roots of couch grass and peppermint); the vegetable juice mix. No water.

Do not cut out the small amount of oil and butter, even though they may appear fattening; they are essential because some vitamins and minerals cannot be absorbed without them.

Applications

Ivy is an ingredient in many creams and has a noticeable effect on cellulite when used on its own. It can be crushed and rubbed into the skin or applied as a compress. Take two handfuls of common ivy, leaves and stalks, boil for 10–15 minutes. When tepid soak cotton pads in the liquid, place between two pieces of gauze and put on areas of cellulite, bandaging firmly into place. Leave for 20 minutes.

Firming Lotion

To firm the flabby skin that often results from weight or cellulite reduction, rub this lotion over the skin in a friction manner at least once a day: pre-boil a litre of water so that the minerals precipitate and can be strained off; when the water is tepid, add 10 g. each of lavender flowers, nettles and lesser celandine leaves. Leave to steep for 24 hours, filter, use. Don't make more than a litre at a time; it is more effective freshly made.

The three parts of this plan work together to help disperse cellulite. It does, however, require patience; the average time for appreciable results is four weeks.

LEGS AND FEET

FLAKY SKIN

Often a winter complaint; apart from keeping your legs well creamed, try the following treatments.

Honey: Splash warm water on legs, rub in a good layer of honey; leave from 20 to 30 minutes to be thoroughly absorbed by the skin; rinse off the honey with warm water, pat dry. Use daily until the condition improves.

Olive cream: Melt together, in a bowl standing in simmering water, 2 tablespoons olive oil and 2 tablespoons lanolin. Mix very well and leave to cool. Apply a very thin film to the legs and massage in thoroughly. Again a daily treatment.

SWOLLEN ANKLES

Because it is mostly a matter of fluid retention, follow the cellulite diet and drink the herbal tea prescribed. Frequently bathe the feet and ankles in warm water with Epsom salts; try ivy compresses.

FEET

Feet suffer from fatigue, dryness, hardened skin and sometimes blisters. Try these treatments.

Epsom salts: Bathe tired feet in a quart (1 l.) of lukewarm water to which 2 tablespoons of Epsom salts have been added; then immerse them in cold water, rub with alcohol and moisturize.

Sea-salt and herbs: Prepare two bowls, one with hot water containing a cup of sea-salt, the other with cold water containing an infusion of rosemary and lavender. Put feet in the hot water for 5 minutes, then in the cold for 1 minute; back to the hot for 5 minutes, back to the cold for 1. Again in the hot for 5 (add hot water if it has cooled). Scrub to thin the skin and then dip the feet briefly in the cold water. This revives and thoroughly cleans.

Mustard powder: To warm up cold or wet feet, put a pinch of mustard in a bowl of hot water and soak the feet for 10 minutes.

Cloves: For aching feet. Thoroughly rub in a mixture of 3 tablespoons sesame oil with 4 drops oil of clove.

Lavender oil: For tired feet. A few drops of lavender oil in a tepid foot bath.

Lemon juice: Softens the skin and revives aching feet.

Yogurt: Softens the skin. Stir 1 teaspoon malt vinegar into a small carton of natural yogurt; brush all over the feet, soles, heels, between the toes; leave for 5 minutes, rinse off.

Cornstarch: Helps blisters. Dab on.

Foot Cream
3 tablespoons lanolin
$1\frac{1}{2}$ tablespoons almond oil
$1\frac{1}{2}$ tablespoons glycerine
2 drops oil of rose geranium

Melt the lanolin in a double boiler or a glass bowl standing in hot water; add the almond oil, glycerine and oil of rose geranium; beat well.

Foot Powder (cooling)
$\frac{1}{2}$ teaspoon menthol
$1\frac{1}{2}$ teaspoons witch hazel
1 teaspoon boric acid powder
7 oz. (200 g.) powdered or precipitated chalk

Dissolve the menthol in the witch hazel, add to the mixture of boric acid powder and chalk; stir until powder has absorbed all the liquid; sift several times.

Corns and Callouses
A hot foot bath containing 2 tablespoons bicarbonate of soda helps soften corns and callouses. After drying, rub in a mixture of $\frac{1}{4}$ cup of oil and 2 teaspoons vinegar.

HANDS

Hands require constant care and protection:
   Milk: Helps chapped rough hands; each night soak in a bowl of cold or warm milk for 5 minutes.
   Vinegar: Rinsing the hands in a mild solution of cider vinegar and water after washing, removes harmful alkaline effects, keeps the hands soft and protects them against drying and chapping.
   Oatmeal or bran: An excellent substitute for soap; keep a bowl near the wash basin, moisten the hands, dip in, rub thoroughly to clean and rinse.
   Lemon: A slice of lemon, or its juice, will get rid of stubborn dirt.
   Cucumber: Combine the juice with an equal quantity of witch hazel for chapped hands.
   Sugar: Cleans stained hands when mixed in equal proportions with sesame or sunflower oil.

Protection Cream (when doing heavy work)
2 teaspoons fuller's earth
2 teaspoons almond oil
2 egg yolks

Mix all three ingredients together into an even blend – it will be like a paste; chill until use. Keep on during work, preferably under gloves.

Night Cream (to be worn under gloves)
3 tablespoons lanolin
1 tablespoon sesame oil

Melt the oils together in a double boiler, blend well and allow to cool. Rub well into the hands.

Almond Night Cream (to be worn under gloves)
2 egg yolks
2 teaspoons rice flour (or ground almonds)
4 teaspoons almond oil
1 tablespoon rose water
$\frac{1}{2}$ teaspoon benzoin

Beat the egg yolks, blend in the rice flour, slowly add the almond oil and rose water – if too stiff, add a little more rose water; then drop by drop add the benzoin. It is quite a thick cream. Pat on the hands; rinse without using soap.

Potato Hand Cream
2 potatoes, medium size
1 tablespoon almond oil
1 tablespoon glycerine
1 teaspoon orange flower water

Cook and mash the potatoes, add the oils and finally the orange flower water; if too thick add extra orange flower water. It makes a paste rather than a cream. Allow to nourish hands for an hour; rinse off.

Orange Hand Jelly
1 tablespoon glycerine
1 tablespoon arrowroot
5 tablespoons orange flower water

Heat the glycerine in a double boiler, slowly add the arrowroot and mix to form a paste; in another pot warm the orange flower water, add to the paste and stir until the mixture clears; use more or less orange flower water to control consistency.

Honey Hand Cream
6 oz. (170 g.) lanolin
3 oz. (85 g.) honey
3 oz. (85 g.) almond oil

Melt the lanolin in a double boiler, allow to cool slightly, add the honey and whisk to blend (by hand or in a blender), then fold in the almond oil and beat until smooth.

Almond Day Cream
3 oz. (85 g.) ground almonds
$\frac{1}{4}$ pint (1·5 dl.) milk
1 egg yolk
2 teaspoons almond oil

Simmer the almonds in the milk until it has all been absorbed; beat the egg yolk and stir it in; bring mixture to the boil for a minute or two. Cool, then fold in the almond oil.

NAILS

To Strengthen

Soak fingertips in an infusion of dill or horsetail daily for 10 minutes.
    Paint nails with white iodine after each immersion in water.
    Mix equal parts castor oil and glycerine and rub into fingertips and cuticles.
    Dip finger nails in apple cider vinegar nightly for 5 minutes.

To Nourish

2 teaspoons beaten egg yolk, 2 teaspoons almond oil, 2 teaspoons honey – mix together and massage into the nails (only a thin film is needed). Leave overnight.

To Colour

Make a paste with henna powder and warm water, using a teaspoon of henna and slowly adding the water until a firm paste is achieved; rub over nails, leave until dry and rinse off; the nails should be pink tinged.

Cuticle Softener

2 tablespoons fresh or frozen pineapple juice

2 tablespoons egg yolk

$\frac{1}{2}$ teaspoon cider vinegar

Mix together. It makes a very sloppy mixture in which the nails should be soaked for 30 minutes; it should be kept in the refrigerator.

TEETH

Cleansers

Apple juice: Dip a brush in the fresh juice and use.

Strawberry: Helps remove stains, rub the fresh fruit over the teeth.

Sage: The fresh leaves rubbed over the teeth and gums cleanse well.

Vinegar: Apple cider vinegar – 1 teaspoon in $\frac{1}{2}$ glass of water – taken after each meal helps to reduce plaque and whitens teeth.

Bicarbonate of soda: This cleans but does not wear away the teeth; use half a teaspoon each time on a dampened brush.

Gum myrrh: Add to the bicarbonate of soda to refresh and tone the gums. To each half pound (225 g.) of bicarbonate of soda, add 6 teaspoons gum myrrh.

MOUTH

Refreshing Washes

Mint: An infusion of 1 part mint to 2 parts water

Cornflowers: A decoction of 1 part to 2 parts water.

Bicarbonate of soda: In a glass of water put one teaspoon bicarbonate of soda and one teaspoon salt.

Cloves: Chew a couple.

Parsley: Chew fresh leaves, or dilute an infusion with equal parts water.

LIPS

Soothing Balm (for chapped or dry lips)

$1\frac{1}{2}$ oz. (45 g.) beeswax

1 oz. (30 g.) honey

2 oz. (60 g.) sesame oil

Melt the beeswax in a double boiler, blend in the honey and then the oil, whisking to a smooth consistency.

Lip Gloss
½ teaspoon beeswax
2 tablespoons cocoa butter

Melt wax and add the cocoa butter; it will solidify on cooling and can be applied with a brush.

Coloured Lip Gloss (pink to burgundy)
1 tablespoon beeswax
5 tablespoons sesame oil
alkanet root colouring

Melt the beeswax and the oil in a container in boiling water; just before pouring into small jars add the colouring – see page 189 on the process of obtaining colour from alkanet; the depth of colour is controlled by the amount you add.

EYES

For Tired Eyes

Witch hazel: Soak pads in witch hazel, close the eyelids and place the pads over them; lie down for half an hour; be careful not to let the liquid enter the eyes.

Herbal infusion: Make a mild infusion of parsley, camomile, fennel or coltsfoot; when tepid, use as an eye wash.

Cucumber: Place a fresh slice over each closed eye; or squeeze the juice from ¼ cucumber and use as an eye bath.

Cold tea: Steep 2 teabags in cold water, squeeze out excess liquid and place over the eyelids; keep on for 10 minutes, lying down.

For Inflamed, Bloodshot Eyes

Borage: Use compresses dipped into borage infusion – 1 teaspoon of the dried herb to a cup of boiling water (or a handful of the fresh herb); allow to cool; place on closed eyes for 10 minutes. This also helps eyes that water a lot.

Camomile: Compresses dipped in a camomile infusion will brighten the eyes and ease strain. Use 1 teaspoon of the dried herb to a cup of boiling water; cool; or steep 2 teabags in hot water; leave on the eyes for 10 minutes.

Goldenseal: Compresses of the infusion; mix half a teaspoon of the powdered herb in a cup of hot water; leave on eyes for 15 minutes, re-dipping compresses when they dry out.

For Under-Eye Puffiness

Potato: Grate a raw potato and put a teaspoonful or two on muslin squares to cover both the lid and under-eye area of closed eye. Leave on for 15 minutes, splash with cold water.

Rose hip: Compresses dipped in a rose hip tisane, either 1 teaspoon in a cup of hot water or 2 teabags. Leave on for 15 minutes.

Papaya: Steep 2 teabags in a cup of boiling water; while still warm place on eye area and leave for 10 minutes.

Fig: Halve a fresh fig and put a piece under each eye; leave for 15 minutes.

Witch hazel: Make the witch hazel water very cold in the refrigerator; soak cottonwool pads, leave on the eyes for 15 minutes.

For Lines Around Eyes

Oil: Lubricate morning and night with a few drops of almond or coconut oil; very gentle movements with fingertips. If possible, give an all-night treatment of cottonwool pads soaked in warm almond or coconut oil; pads can be held in place with a sleeping mask or a wide bandage.

Egg white: A temporary measure that will smooth the eye area for a few hours. The drying effect of the egg white tightens under-eye tissue and gives a smooth appearance; pat on a very thin film of unbeaten white of an egg, better still brush it on with a paint brush – the thinner the coating the more effective; allow the egg white to dry and then apply make-up, but pat it on with the fingertips instead of smoothing. After removing the make-up, oil the eye area well, because egg white is very drying.

Eye Make-up Remover

2 tablespoons almond oil (or coconut oil)
1 tablespoon castor oil

Mix the oils together well; remove make-up with a cottonwool pad.

EYELASHES

Castor oil will slowly improve the condition of weak or short lashes, but it can take months - apply nightly.

EYEBROWS

Warm olive oil can sometimes encourage growth – rub into the eyebrows nightly, in the direction of growth.

HAIR

Ideally hair should be immaculately clean and glossy with a bounce that makes it a living part of your body.

Good condition of hair depends on care and attention and is even more important than styling.

Condition is basically determined by genes and what you eat. A high-protein diet with lots of fresh fruit and vegetables is good for hair – protein meaning not more meat, but more fish, cheese, eggs, milk, nuts, protein vegetables and grains. Foods containing vitamins of the B complex are essential, particularly pantothenic acid and the PABA group. Of the minerals, iron, iodine and copper are beneficial, while lack of iodine can be very detrimental. A supplement of brewer's yeast tablets and large daily helpings of wheatgerm are recommended for anyone with a hair problem. It has also been said that grey hair can be helped by large doses of vitamin B.

Dry hair should be washed weekly and given a conditioning treatment every three weeks; oily hair should be washed as frequently as necessary, dry shampooed at times and conditioned once a month. Balanced hair needs washing weekly and conditioning once a month. Any type of bleached, lightened, tinted or permed hair needs conditioning more frequently, particularly in the case of dry hair made even drier by chemical alteration.

SHAMPOOS

Mild Shampoo
$\frac{1}{2}$ oz. (15 g.) crushed soapwort root
2 pints (1 l.) boiling water

Make an infusion of the soapwort, steeping it in the hot water for 15 minutes; strain. Half a cup is needed to shampoo hair.

Simple Soap Shampoo

4 oz. (100 g.) old-fashioned green soap (or home-made soap, see page 187)

1 pint (6 dl.) warm water

Grate the soap and dissolve in the water; it may take a few days to coagulate evenly. Stir frequently. Use in small quantities.

Mild Herbal Shampoo

½ oz. (15 g.) crushed soapwort root

½ oz. (15 g.) camomile flowers or rosemary

2 pints (1 l.) boiling water

Put the soapwort and the herbs together in a bowl and cover with the hot water to make an infusion; leave for 15 minutes, strain before use; a cupful is sufficient for one shampoo. Alternatively, a strong infusion of camomile or rosemary can be added to a castile shampoo.

Egg Yolk Shampoo

2 egg yolks

1 cup warm water

Beat the yolks into the water; massage into the scalp and through the hair for 5 minutes; leave to soak in for 10 minutes. Rinse off – no other shampooing is necessary.

Egg and Brandy Shampoo

½ cup warm water

½ cup brandy

2 egg yolks

Combine the water and brandy, slowly beat in the egg yolks; massage into hair; allow 10 minutes for complete absorption; rinse away.

Egg and Orange Shampoo

½ oz. (15 g.) crushed soapwort root

1 pint (6 dl.) boiling water

1 egg yolk

1 tablespoon orange juice

Make an infusion of the soapwort and boiling water and leave to steep for 15 minutes; strain. Combine the egg yolk and orange juice, then beat into the infusion. Massage into the hair, and leave for 10 minutes; rinse.

Egg and Camomile Shampoo (light hair only)
(for dry hair)
1 cup strong camomile infusion
1 egg yolk

(for oily hair)
1 cup strong camomile infusion
1 egg white

Beat either the yolk or the white of the egg (depending on hair) into the infusion.

Sage or Rosemary and Egg Shampoo   This is for dark hair, using exactly the same recipe as above, but substituting a sage or rosemary infusion for that of camomile.

Oily Hair Shampoo
4 whole eggs
1 cup rum
1 cup rose water

First beat the eggs, massage through hair, leave for 15 minutes; rinse off well with water.

    Now mix the rum and rose water together, using this as a rinse; pour through the hair two or three times.

Anti-Dandruff Shampoo
2 egg yolks
$\frac{1}{2}$ cup warm water
2 teaspoons apple cider vinegar
1 cup tepid water

Beat the egg yolks into the warm water, massage into scalp and hair, leave for 10 minutes, rinse with warm water.

    Combine the apple cider vinegar and tepid water and rinse through the hair two or three times.

Dry Shampoo
orris-root

Sprinkle a small amount through the hair and brush for 5 minutes, or mix the following powders together and use in the same way:
$\frac{1}{4}$ oz. (7 g.) orris-root powder
$\frac{1}{4}$ oz. (7 g.) arrowroot powder

CONDITIONERS

Simple Treatments

Olive oil: Good for brittle, dry hair. Warm 2 tablespoons of olive oil, gently massage into every part of the scalp and comb through. Then wrap the head in a steaming towel. Treat for 20 to 30 minutes, reheating the towel if necessary. Shampoo and rinse.

Castor oil: Good for fragile hair and broken ends; warm $\frac{1}{2}$ cup of castor oil, massage into the scalp and comb through; wind a steaming towel around the head and leave for 30 minutes before shampooing.

Avocado: Nourishing for all hair. Mash a whole avocado, massage into the hair and scalp, cover with a plastic bag and leave for an hour before shampooing.

Recipes for Conditioners

The following are conditioning formulas; they should all be well massaged into the hair, combed through and left on for 20 to 30 minutes; the hair has to be covered with a plastic bag to encourage and retain heat. All are for application before shampooing unless otherwise stated.

Egg and Honey Conditioner
1 teaspoon honey
2 teaspoons sesame or safflower oil
1 egg
Combine the honey and oil in a double boiler. When blended beat the egg and slowly stir in until an even consistency is achieved.

Olive Oil and Honey Conditioner
$\frac{1}{2}$ cup olive oil (the greener the better)
1 cup liquid honey
Stir together, put in a jar and shake well; leave to steep for a day or two, shaking every so often. For dark hair.

Cocoa Butter Conditioner
1 tablespoon cocoa butter
1 tablespoon lanolin
$\frac{1}{2}$ cup safflower oil

Melt all three in a double boiler and when completely dissolved and blended take off the heat and beat. For use, add 1 tablespoon of water to 3 tablespoons of the mixture. Good for dark hair.

Protein Conditioner
2 eggs
1 tablespoon olive oil
1 tablespoon glycerine
1 teaspoon cider vinegar

Beat the eggs, slowly add the olive oil, then the glycerine and finally the vinegar. This should be used after an initial shampoo. After using the conditioner, shampoo and rinse again. A restorer for all types of hair.

Coconut Oil Conditioner
2 tablespoons coconut oil
1 egg
1 tablespoon cider vinegar

Melt the coconut oil, beat the egg and blend it in and then add the vinegar. Keep warm otherwise the coconut oil will solidify. Cover the head with a steaming towel.

Conditioner for Gloss
1 oz. (30 g.) beeswax
1 lb. (450 g.) honey
¼ cup almond oil
¼ cup lavender oil
2 tablespoons infusion of thyme

Melt the wax, honey, and oils in a double boiler and slowly add the thyme infusion. Leave on hair for only 15 minutes.

RINSING

After rinsing thoroughly with water, a final natural rinse can often enhance colour and shine.

For All Hair

  Nettle: Improves natural colouring and gives the hair body. Simmer a handful of nettles in a pint (6 dl.) of water until soft; strain and dilute with equal parts water for the final rinse.

Herb infusions: 2 tablespoons of the herb is covered with 1 pint (6 dl.) boiling water and allowed to steep for 30 minutes; strain and use.

horsetail and sage – add shine, improve colour

parsley and catnip – add shine, promote growth

elder flower, lime flower or quince peel – help to prevent dandruff and bring a shine.

Comb-out Lotion

(makes hair silky and smooth)

2 tablespoons rosemary (for dark hair)

or

2 tablespoons camomile (for light hair)

1 pint (6 dl.) boiling water

3 oz. (90 g.) almond oil

20 drops lavender essence

Pour boiling water over the herb, steep for 30 minutes, strain; add the almond oil and finally lavender essence.

For Dark Hair

Vinegar: $\frac{1}{2}$ cup apple cider vinegar in a quart (1 l.) of water gives shine and body to hair.

Rosemary or lemon verbena: An infusion – 2 tablespoons covered with 1 pint (6 dl.) boiling water, steep for 30 minutes; adds shine, helps bring out colour and highlights.

For Fair Hair

Lemon juice: Add 1 teaspoon to the last rinsing water.

Camomile: To restore light tones to blond hair simmer a cup of dried camomile flowers in a pint (6 dl.) of water for 15 minutes, strain; use as a final rinse, pouring it through the hair several times.

Rhubarb root: To lighten hair. Simmer 4 tablespoons of ground rhubarb root in $1\frac{1}{2}$ pints (9 dl.) water for 30 minutes and steep for several hours; strain and rinse through hair two or three times.

TO HELP DANDRUFF

Apple: Make a liquid of 1 part apple juice to 3 parts water; rub into the scalp two or three times a week.

Nettle: Make a strong infusion of nettles (by boiling the leaves in water until soft – takes about 30 minutes); to $\frac{1}{2}$ cup of this add 2 tablespoons apple cider vinegar; massage into the scalp morning and evening.

Rosemary: To $\frac{1}{2}$ cup rosemary infusion add a pinch of boric acid powder; massage daily into the scalp.

COLOURING

Natural hair colourants are limited and often unpredictable to work with. Apart from henna, the other dyes and bleaches need many applications before visible changes are observed. Results depend a lot on the type of hair, its condition and original colour.

Henna

The strongest natural colourant, giving various shades of red according to the strength, treatment time and type of hair. It is completely non-toxic (and can therefore be used on pubic hair). It is, however, slightly astringent, so it is best to rub the skin with oil before applying henna. The colour lasts several months.

It must be used with caution because controlling colour without experience is difficult. It is very easy to be left with fearsome shades of red. A patch test is an absolute necessity, whether it is used alone or in combination with other vegetable dyes. The hair must be shampooed before using henna; wear gloves so as not to dye the hands as well. Shades of mahogany, auburn and red can be achieved.

Basic Henna Formula
2 cups henna powder
1 cup warm water
1 teaspoon vinegar

Mix the powder and water into a thick paste and add the vinegar, which helps to release the dye. Allow to stand for an hour. Put in a double boiler, heat until well warmed; leave for half an hour.

Brush on to the hair in sections; comb through very thoroughly. Wrap the head in plastic or a towel. The final colour depends on the length of time the henna is left on the hair. For mahogany tones you will need about three hours, for reddish tones longer. But keep on checking – once the colour takes it is permanent; checks should be made every 30 minutes. When the colour is right, wash the hair and keep rinsing until water is clear, combing all the time.

Henna and Sage

This provides a more subtle shade than henna, more auburn.

$\frac{1}{2}$ cup dried sage

1 pint (6 dl.) boiling water

1 tablespoon henna

1 teaspoon ground cloves

Steep the sage in the boiling water and leave overnight. Mix together the henna and cloves; add enough of the sage infusion to make a malleable paste. Distribute through the clean freshly shampooed hair and comb; cover the head with plastic or a towel. Leave the colour to develop for 30 minutes before the first check; if a deeper tone is wanted leave it longer, but check constantly.

Henna and Camomile

This brings lighter reddish tones to fading brown hair.

$\frac{1}{2}$ cup dried camomile flowers

1 pint (6 dl.) boiling water

1 tablespoon henna

1 teaspoon vinegar

Steep the camomile flowers in the boiling water overnight; add the vinegar. Put the henna powder in a bowl and slowly pour in the liquid, stirring all the time, until a paste is formed. Test for colour 30 minutes after application.

Other Colourants

Camomile   Traditionally a bleaching agent and lightener in both paste and liquid form. To make the bleaching paste, first prepare a strong infusion of camomile flowers and leave overnight; add enough kaolin powder to form a paste. The hair has to be shampooed first. The paste should be left on for an hour, the head being swathed in plastic or towelling. Finally rinse off with warm water.

You may be disappointed at the first result, but with repeated use, this paste is more effective.

Walnut
This darkens hair within the brown shades.
6 tablespoons green walnut skins
2 tablespoons alum powder
$\frac{1}{2}$ cup orange flower water

Chop up the walnut skins very finely, grind as thoroughly as possible and then mix with the alum powder. Add enough orange flower water to make a firm paste. Put the paste on the hair before washing and leave for about an hour, but check after 30 minutes. Rinse off, then shampoo.

Rhubarb Root
An effective lightener for dark blond hair; it can also give rich, golden hues to brown hair.
$\frac{1}{2}$ cup crushed rhubarb root
$1\frac{1}{2}$ pints (9 dl.) water

Simmer the root in water for 20–30 minutes; steep for 3 hours; strain. To make a paste add $\frac{1}{2}$ cup of kaolin powder to 1 cup of the decoction. Apply the paste to the hair for varying times from 15 minutes to 1 hour, depending on the degree of lightness required.

Tea and Sage
The following is a recipe said to help counteract grey hair. It should be rubbed into the hair, particularly at the roots, four or five times a week.
1 tablespoon Indian tea
1 tablespoon dried sage
1 tablespoon rum
$3\frac{1}{2}$ pints (2 l.) water

Simmer the tea and the sage in water for $1\frac{1}{2}$–2 hours; strain and cool. Add the rum, shaking well before use.

Colour Rinses

These can give slight colour changes; use these herbal infusions as a final rinse, pouring through hair two or three times.

Marigold flowers: Give reddish tints; steep $\frac{1}{2}$ cup of marigold flowers in 1 pint (6 dl.) boiling water and leave overnight; use after straining.

Saffron: Again for reddish tints. Put a pinch of saffron in a cup of boiling water, stir well and leave until tepid; rinse through the hair.

Camomile: Lightens hair – $\frac{1}{2}$ cup dried flowers steeped in 1 pint (6 dl.) boiling water overnight.

Privet: Chestnut highlights for brown hair; $\frac{1}{2}$ cup of privet leaves steeped overnight in 1 pint (6 dl.) boiling water. For a lighter chestnut, add 2 teaspoons of quince juice to the infusion.

Sage: Made into a rinse that is dabbed on each day, not put through the hair all at once. It helps bring brown tones to grey hair. Half a cup of sage is steeped overnight in 1 pint (6 dl.) boiling water; make a cup of strong Indian tea, allowing it to steep for 30 minutes; combine the two liquids and boil together for half an hour; steep for 3 hours. Dab it into the hair daily.

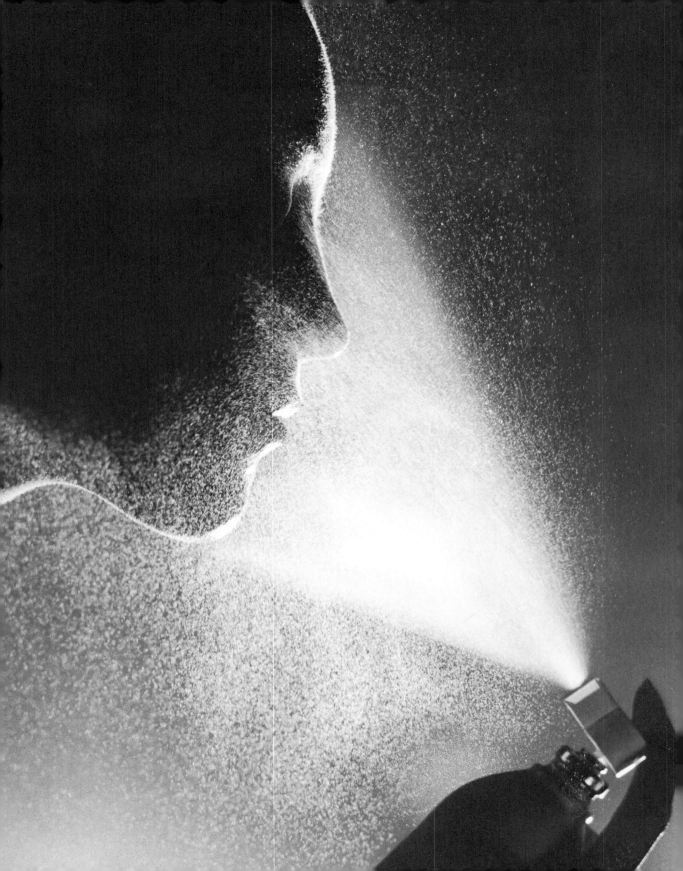

4

FRAGRANCES

Most great perfumes are a combination of natural essences and oils, but amateurs cannot attempt complex and subtle blendings. Fragrances developed on your own involve simple formulas, using well-known flowers and essential oils to make colognes, sachets and potpourris.

Lavender Toilet Water
$\frac{1}{2}$ oz. (15 g.) oil of lavender
2 pints (1 l.) ethyl alcohol (or 80° proof vodka)
2 teaspoons rose water

Mix the lavender oil with a little alcohol until blended, then slowly add the remainder; finally stir in the rose water. Keep in sealed jars; mature for 6 weeks before use.

Cologne Water
$1\frac{1}{2}$ teaspoons oil of lavender
1 teaspoon orange flower water
1 teaspoon lemon essence
1 teaspoon bergamot
1 pint (6 dl.) ethyl alcohol

Blend all the oils and essences and then gradually mix in the alcohol. Allow to mature for 6–8 weeks; keep in stoppered glass bottles.

Floral Cologne
$3\frac{1}{2}$ teaspoons oil of lavender
$\frac{1}{2}$ oz. (15 g.) oil of cloves
6 oz. (180 g.) ethyl alcohol
1 oz. (30 g.) rose water

Blend the two oils with a little alcohol until well mixed: beat in the remaining alcohol. Add the rose water. Bottle tightly and mature for 6–8 weeks.

Herb and Flower Cologne
¼ oz. (7 g.) bergamot
¼ oz. (7 g.) thyme
¼ oz. (7 g.) orange oil
¼ oz. (7 g.) balsam of Peru
¼ oz. (7 g.) essence of cloves
¼ pint (1.5 dl.) orange flower water
2 pints (1 l.) ethyl alcohol

Put all the herbs and essences into a glass jar, pour over the alcohol slowly and stir constantly. Keep in tightly lidded jars; allow to mature for 2 weeks.

Oriental Cologne
3 drops oil of lavender
10 drops oil of clove
20 drops tincture of musk
1 pint (6 dl.) ethyl alcohol

Put all the essences in a jar, pour over the alcohol very slowly, stirring until completely mixed. Put in lidded jar, shake very well. Leave to mature for 2 weeks.

After-Bath Lotion
3½ oz. (100 g.) red rose petals
2 pints (1 l.) white vinegar

Make in a ceramic jar. Pour vinegar over the petals, cover with muslin and allow to steep for 15 days; strain.

Basic Cream Perfume
½ cup grated beeswax
½ cup almond oil
4 tablespoons water
20 drops any of the above colognes

Melt the wax in a double boiler, beat in the oil very slowly and then add the water. Remove from the heat and stir in the cologne. Whisk until thoroughly blended; pour into small flat jars.

Refreshing Cream Perfume

$\frac{1}{2}$ cup grated beeswax

$\frac{1}{4}$ cup almond oil

2 tablespoons water

20 drops oil of lavender

20 drops oil of musk

10 drops oil of rosemary

10 drops oil of orange

8 drops oil of bergamot

2 drops oil of cloves

Melt the wax in a double boiler, beat in the almond oil and add the water; take off the heat and add all the essences one by one, whisking all the time to distribute the various perfumes evenly. Pour into small flat jars.

POTPOURRIS AND SACHETS

Dried flowers and foliage are used to give clean natural scents. Potpourri mixtures often contain complete petals and leaves, while for the sachets ingredients are finely cut, ground or powdered. A fixative is added, and sometimes an essential oil as well. Potpourris are contained in large glass or china bowls and jars, but they must be lidded. Sachets are small fabric squares (usually of muslin, voile or calico) sewn to contain the mixture.

All the leaves and petals must be absolutely dry before use. They should be gathered in the morning and laid on drying racks. When the materials are completely dry, they should be stored in airtight boxes or jars to await use; keep away from the light to preserve their colour.

Basic Rules

Mixtures are made in a large container and blended for 8 weeks before being transferred to their final bowls or sachets. You can virtually choose your own petals, herbs and spices (though some suggestions follow). First put in the dry material, measuring in a quart (1 l.) jar; then for every quart add 1 tablespoon of fixative (ambergris, civet, musk, benzoin or orris-root). If there are any spices or essential oils in the recipe, add these next. Stir at each step (with a wooden spoon). Put a lid on the container and let the mixture mature for 8 weeks, giving it an occasional stir during that time. Now you can transfer it to decorative containers or sew it into sachets.

You select the ingredients for fragrance, colour and spicy effects. These are the most popular:

Fragrance: acacia, basil, lavender, lemon balm, lemon verbena, marjoram, mint, orange tree leaves, patchouli, rose, rose geranium leaves, rosemary, sandalwood (bark), violet.

Colour: carnation, delphinium, honeysuckle, larkspur, lavender, lilac, marigold, nasturtium, orange blossom, pansy, rose, violet.

Spice: allspice, caraway seeds, cinnamon, cloves, coriander seeds, mace, nutmeg, dried peel of citrus fruits.

Simple Potpourri (or sachet)

1 pint (6 dl.) rosemary leaves

1 pint (6 dl.) lavender leaves and flowers

1 tablespoon orris-root (the fixative)

2 drops oil of rose geranium

The orris-root should be cut in small pieces for a potpourri. If you use this mixture for a sachet it has to be ground to a powder.

Lavender Potpourri (or sachet)

$\frac{1}{2}$ pint (3 dl.) lavender flowers and leaves

$\frac{1}{2}$ pint (3 dl.) rose petals

2 tablespoons crushed cinnamon sticks

1 tablespoon crushed cloves

2 tablespoons gum benzoin (the fixative)

10 drops oil of lavender

5 drops oil of rose geranium

5 drops oil of bergamot

5 drops oil of lemon

2 teaspoons powdered vanilla bean

Rose Bowl

2 pints (1 l.) dried rose petals

2 tablespoons orris-root (the fixative)

2 teaspoons ground allspice

1 teaspoon nutmeg

1 teaspoon crushed cinnamon sticks

1 teaspoon crushed cloves

dried orange and lemon peel

vanilla bean

dried vetiver root

$\frac{1}{2}$ teaspoon rose geranium oil

Mix the first six ingredients together very well, then add little bits of dried orange and lemon peel, vanilla bean, vetiver root. Add $\frac{1}{2}$ teaspoon of rose geranium oil, stir well; add a little lemon verbena oil if it appears on the dry side. Seal the jar for 6 weeks. Open and stir well, add more rose petals if you like. Periodically close the jar for a period of a month, so that the scents can become strong again and permeate the new petals.

Violet Sachet

$\frac{1}{2}$ pint (3 dl.) powdered violet root

2 tablespoons powdered sandalwood

2 drops oil of orange

1 drop oil of lemon

8 drops tincture of musk

Oriental Sachet

$\frac{1}{2}$ pint (3 dl.) patchouli leaves

$\frac{1}{2}$ cup sandalwood (powdered)

2 drops oil of rose geranium

SUN

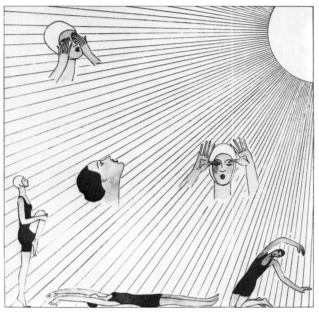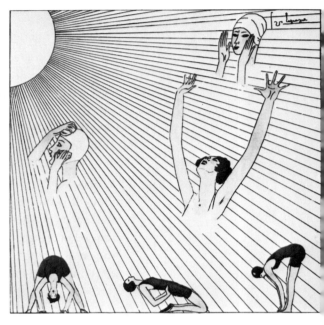

LEPAPE 1927

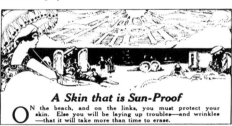

A Skin that is Sun-Proof

ON the beach, and on the links, you must protect your skin. Else you will be laying up troubles—and wrinkles—that it will take more than time to erase.

1921   1921

'Whether to be or not to be sunburned is the question that many women are asking themselves and their beauty specialist, as they leave London to depart for lands of warm skies, to lie on beaches underneath an unaccustomed summer sun, or to play golf bareheaded, in the brilliant light of the South.'

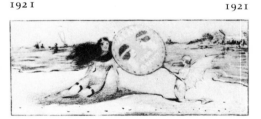

"SHOOING AWAY" FRECKLES *and* SUNBURN

'In days gone by, the thought of the complexion being marred by sunstains, freckles and tan used to cause many women moments of great anxiety . . .

How different it is today, when triumphant science knows how to weave a spell before which freckles and sunstains beat a retreat and by which a clear, diaphanous skin can be maintained through the whole season of summer sports and pastimes.'

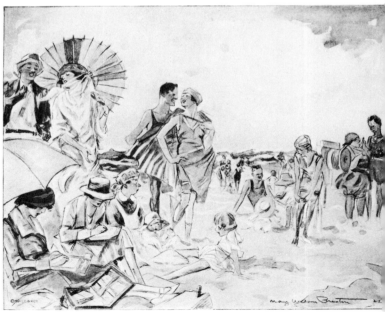

MAY WILSON PRESTON 192

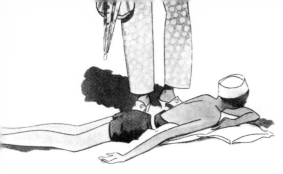

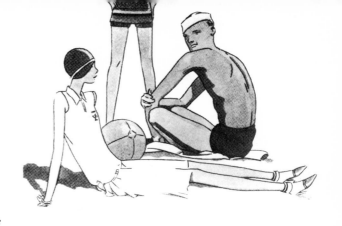

'The lady who is so thorough in her methods of acquiring an even sunburn has a companion in pyjamas with large spots.'
Right, 'The girl wears rolled socks and a jersey dress made to slip over a bathing costume. This year the beret is competing for favour with the white American cap as worn in the United States Navy.'

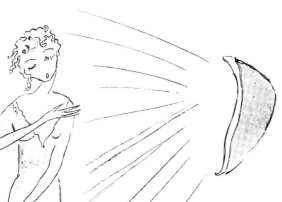

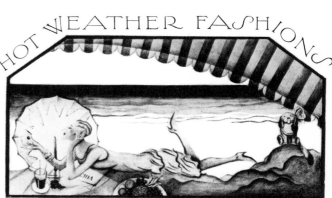

1926

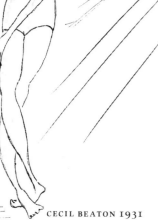

CECIL BEATON 1931

'Thawed and dissolved into a jelly'

'Beer's beach outfit consists of a white cape and jumper covered with black triangles, worn with black shorts and white elasticated belt.'

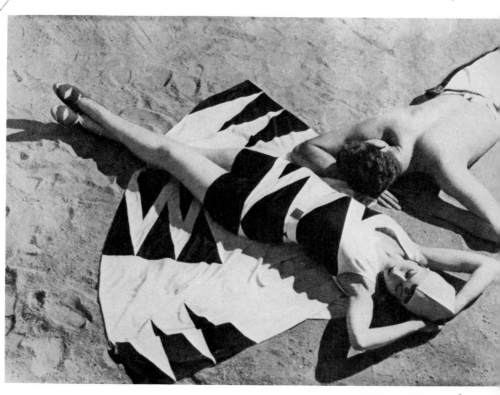

HOYNINGEN-HUENE 1928

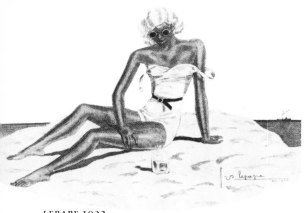

LEPAPE 1932

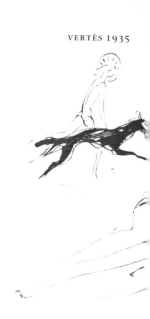

VERTÈS 1935

SCHALL 1934

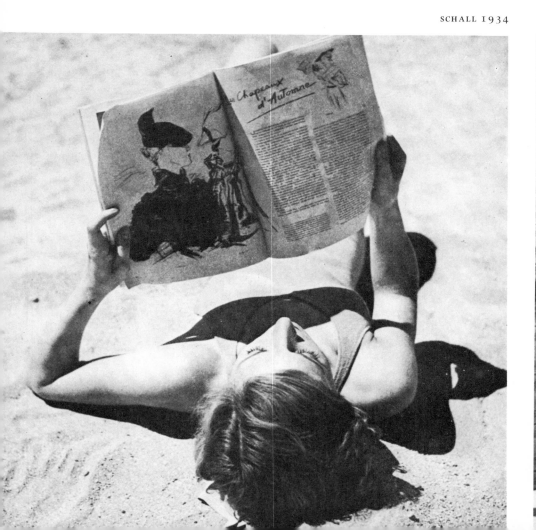

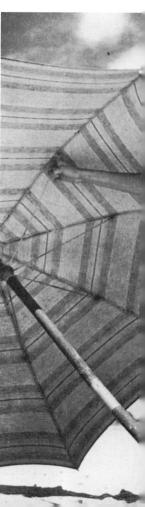

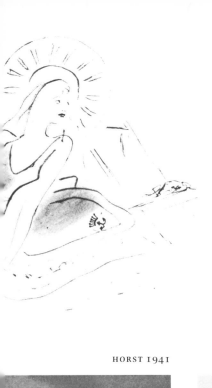

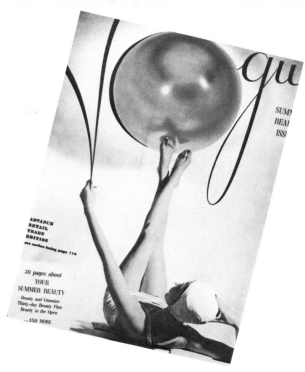

TONI FRISSELL 1941

HORST 1941

COFFIN 1951

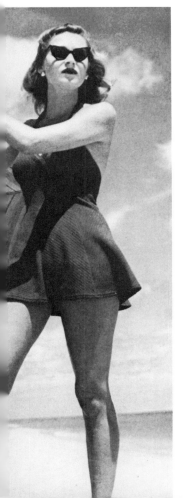

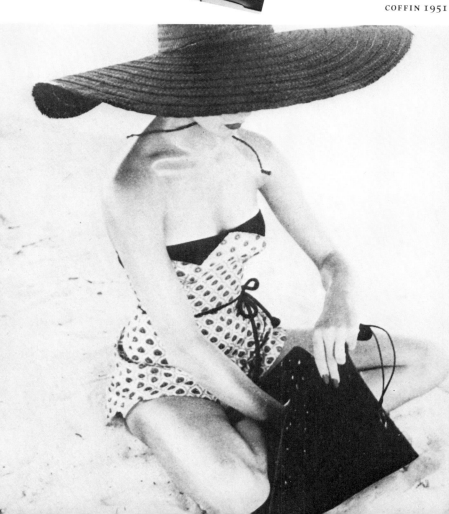

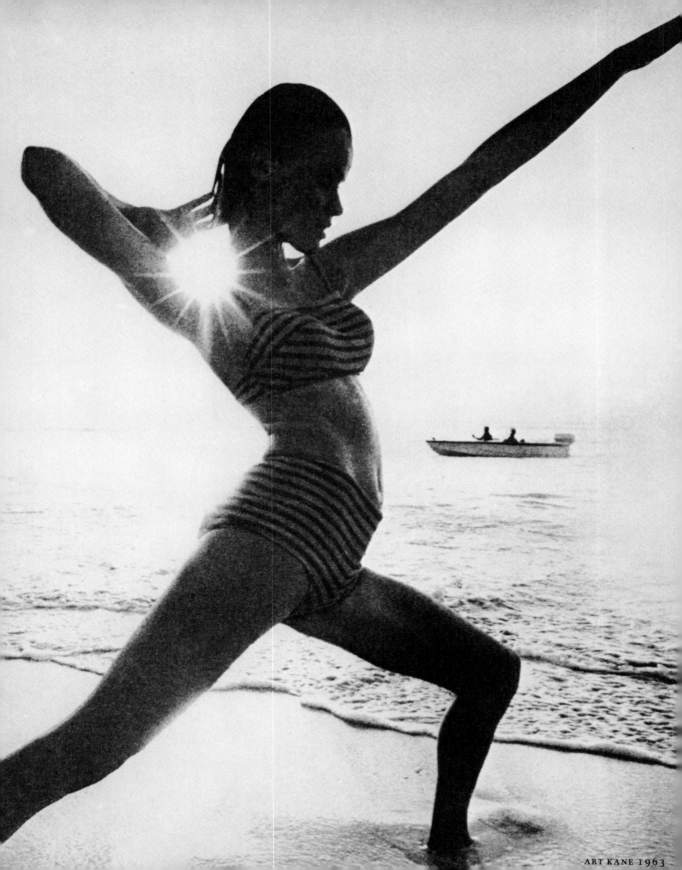

ART KANE 1963

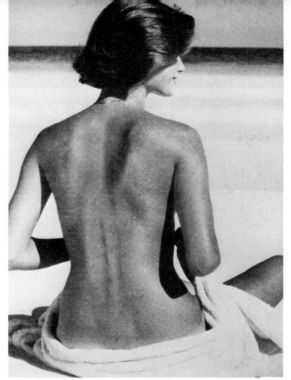

RICO PUHLMANN 1975

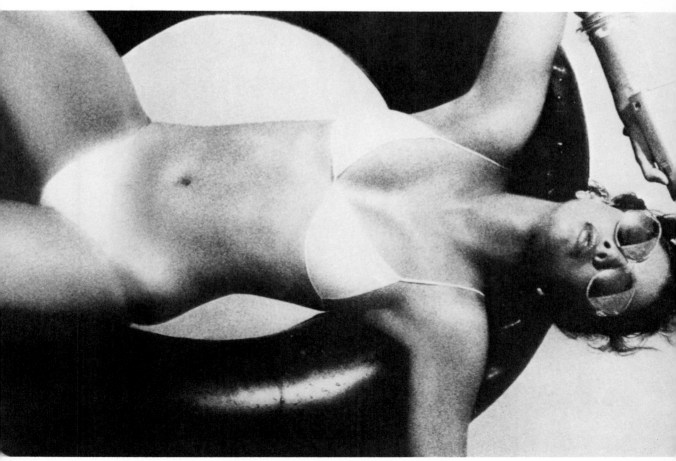

MIKE REINHARDT 1978

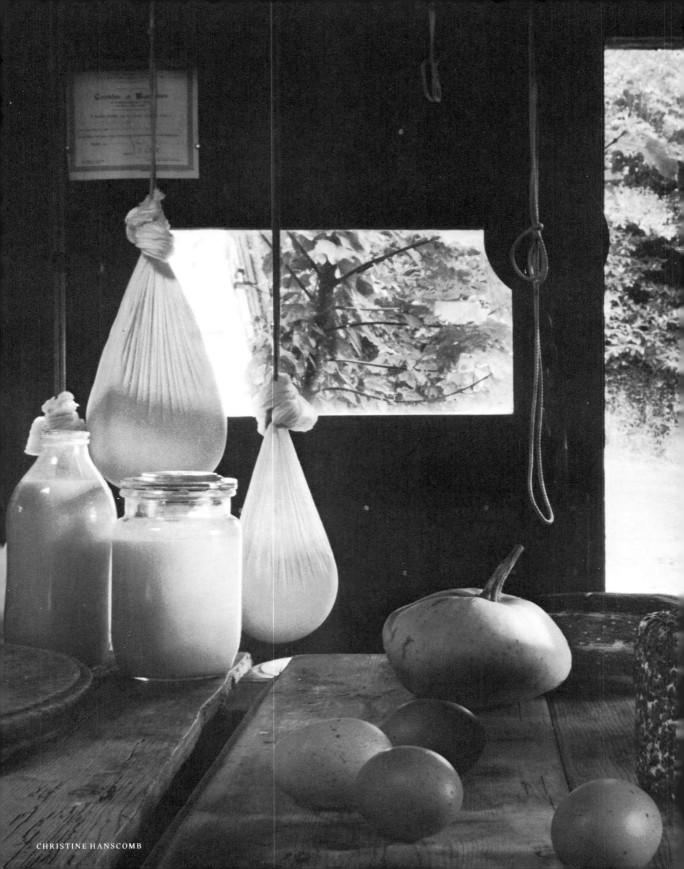

CHRISTINE HANSCOMB

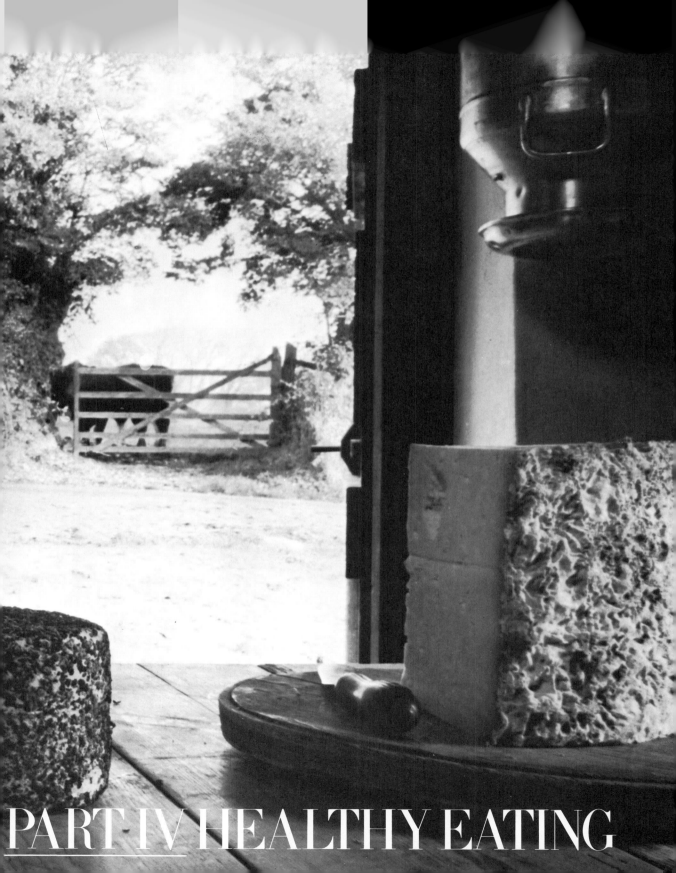

PART IV HEALTHY EATING

1

FOOD VALUES

We get our body-building materials and energy from the food we eat. Good health and vitality depend upon the type and quality of nourishment we get daily. We can help ourselves by careful observance of food values and by being aware of the constructive elements in food. It may seem contradictory when a food according to nutritionists has no specific benefit but in the view of the naturopathic practitioners is a therapeutic aid. That is how it is, so don't be surprised when herbalists praise the very plants that nutritionists belittle. They are looking from different points of view.

Here we are concerned with nutrition. Learning to eat well is basically a matter of becoming aware of the value of specific types of food – grains, vegetables, nuts and so on. It is learning to eat fresh food, to eat more raw foods and to eat less fat and much less sugar. It is rethinking old eating habits in order to reduce meat intake and to eliminate packaged foods; it is learning not to destroy all the goodness in cooking (see page 236).

FOOD GROUPS

The constituents in food can be divided into six groups: protein, carbohydrates, fats, vitamins, minerals and water. The first three indicate function – carbohydrates and fats provide only energy, protein provides nutrients, amino acids and some energy. The vitamin and mineral elements are entirely nutrients, and in some form or other are found in all foods. Water is essential to life, and is contained in all foods in varying amounts.

It is impossible to categorize any food strictly, for all are a mixture, but they are usually listed according to their major function.

Opposite: Tessa Traeger, 1976
Overleaf: Tessa Traeger, 1976, 1977

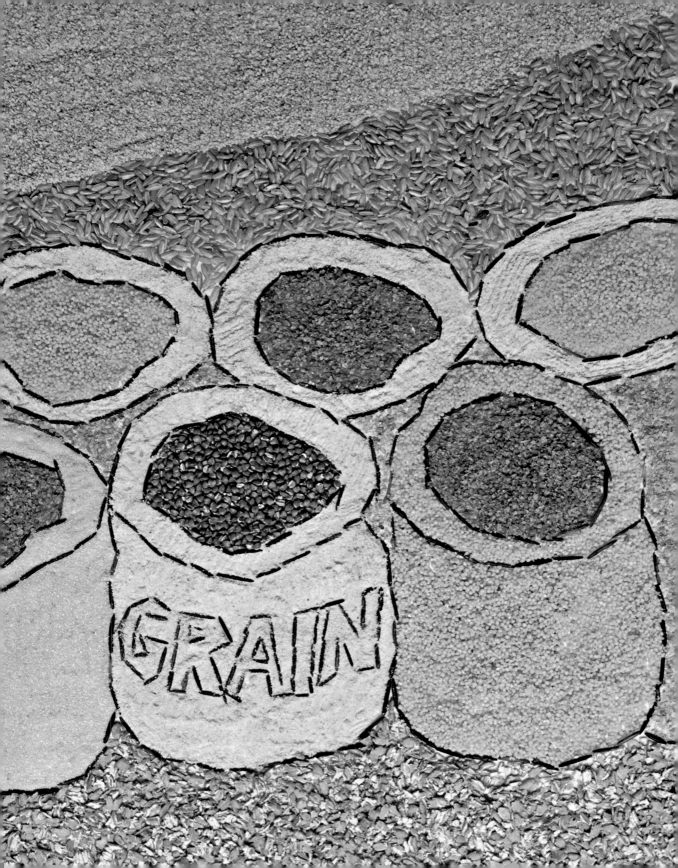

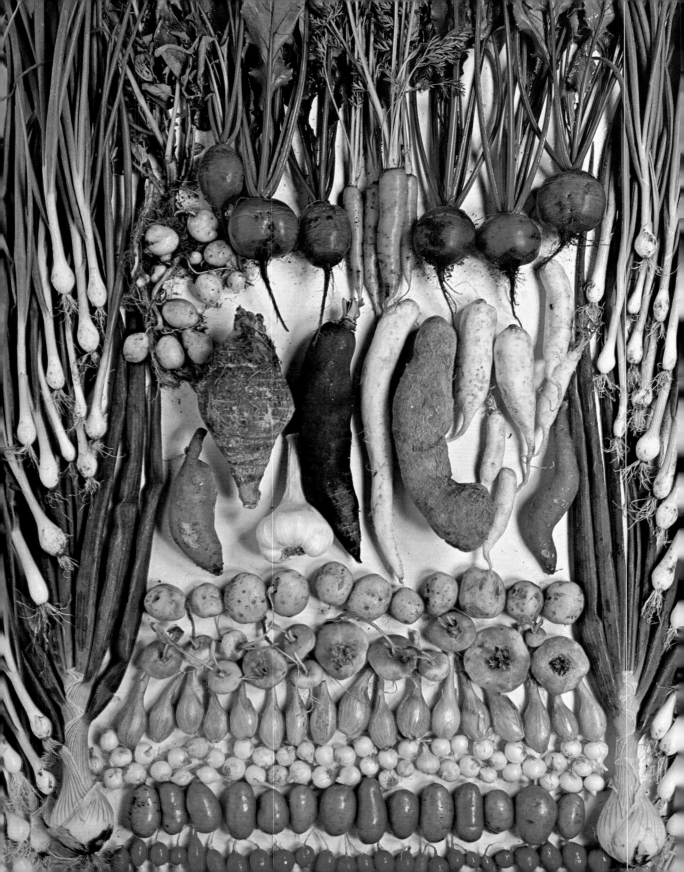

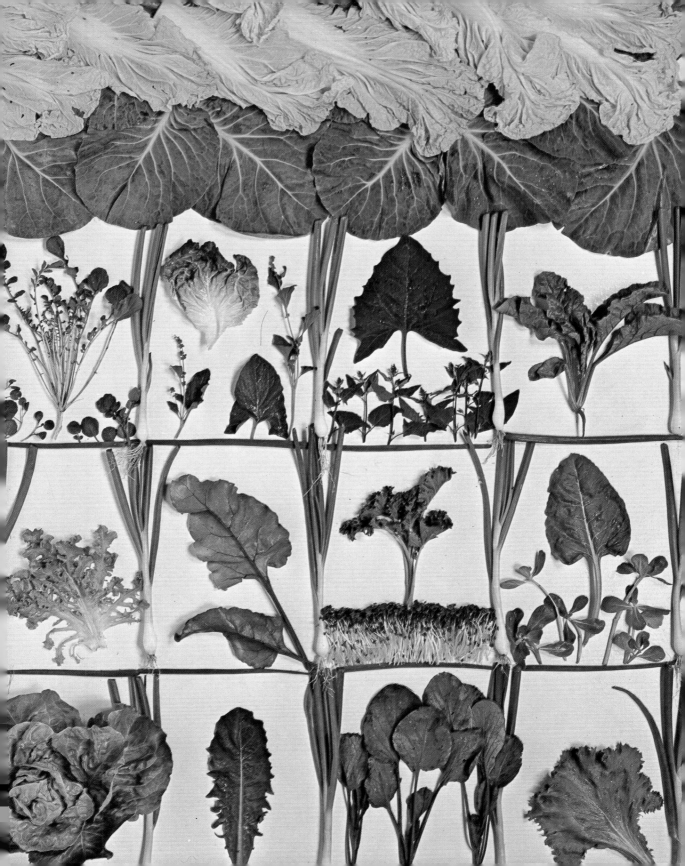

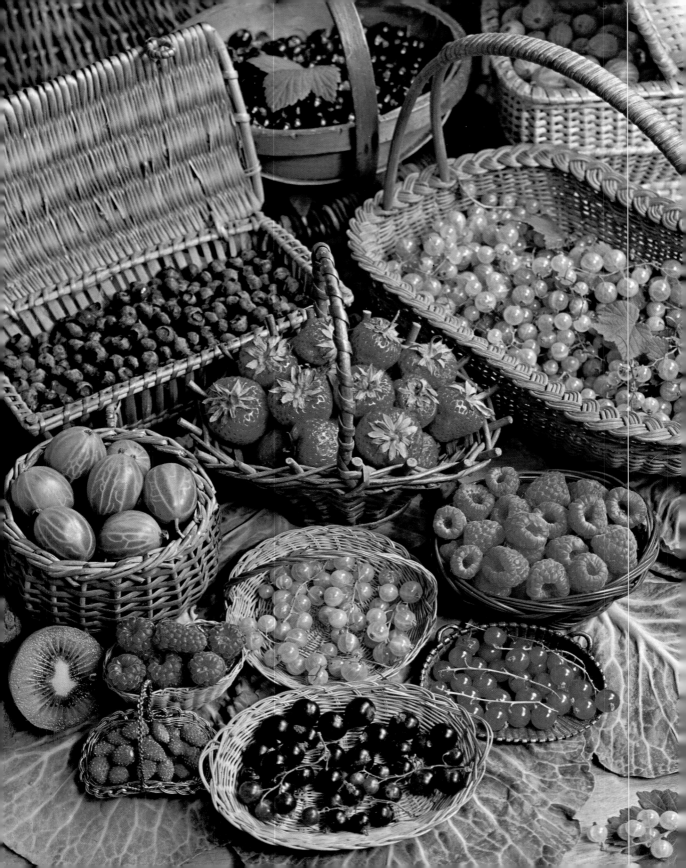

PROTEINS

Mainly for building and repairing body tissue and essential to life. The amino acids in proteins are the significant part and not all proteins contain a full set. In general flesh food, milk and cheese proteins are superior, while the protein in many grains is relatively incomplete. In practice, a diet usually contains many different proteins and what is missing in one is supplied by another. Proteins have so many functions it is impossible to mention them all, but the more important are: the ability to build hormones and enzymes which aid in energy production; digestion of food and excretion from the tissues and body; the making of haemoglobin within the red corpuscles; maintaining the acid-alkaline balance of the body; assisting in clotting the blood; forming antibodies to fight infection.

Proteins are found in flesh foods (meat, fish, poultry), dairy products (eggs, milk, cheese), nuts and seeds, grains and some vegetables.

CARBOHYDRATES

These provide energy for physical and mental activity; they assist in the assimilation and digestion of other foods. There are three types of carbohydrates – sugars, starches and cellulose. The sugars and starches are converted to glucose for energy, and any excess not spent as energy is stored as fat. Ideally, sugar should come from fresh fruits and honey, not from refined table sugar or sweets. Similarly, the refined flours, cereals and breads are a less desirable form of starch carbohydrate. Cellulose carbohydrates (a large part of fruits and vegetables) have no energy value but provide the fibre necessary for digestion. Fibre is the structural part of a plant, the connective tissue that supports the cells, and is the missing ingredient in many diets. It used to be called roughage and was considered essential to the proper working of the bowels. It does not contain nourishment, it passes virtually unchanged through the intestine to be excreted as waste, yet its bulk is necessary to provide a smooth intestinal voyage for other nutrients. It takes a lot of chewing, which produces saliva and gastric juices, aiding in the digestion of other nutrients.

FATS

Fats provide a source of delayed energy and act as carriers for fat-soluble vitamins, particularly important in the case of calcium. They also prevent the skin from becoming dry. It is essential to have fatty deposits protecting vital organs, while a layer under the skin preserves heat and protects the body against cold. A deficiency of fats can lead to a deficiency of vitamins and to skin disorders. Although fat intake should be watched, it should not be cut out. In practice that would in any case be almost impossible; apart from the obvious sources, such as meat, butter, margarine, oils, and so on, fat is also contained in grains and vegetables, nuts, seeds, eggs, milk and cheese. There are two types: saturated fats which are solid at room temperature and come mostly from animal sources; and unsaturated fats, usually liquid and from vegetable sources. From the health point of view, it is considered best to limit animal fats and use mostly vegetable oils such as olive, corn, sunflower, wheatgerm, sesame, avocado and peanut.

VITAMINS

Although not body-builders or forms of energy in themselves, vitamins regulate body function. They help convert fat and carbohydrates into energy; they assist in the repair of tissues; they could be called the incentives of metabolism. Though different vitamins perform quite different functions, they work as a team, which means a deficiency of one may well affect the working of another.

Vitamins are usually called by letters of the alphabet, because when first discovered their composition was unknown. Some nutritionists have now given them chemical names, but they are still commonly referred to by the letters. They fall into two groups: those soluble in fat (A,D,E and K) which enable them to be stored in the body for future use, and those soluble in water (C and B complex) which must be replaced every day as any excess is excreted through the urine or skin evaporation. New vitamins are being discovered and named, but their properties and functions are not fully formulated. It is extremely difficult to test for vitamin deficiency, as only when it is at an advanced stage do visible symptoms occur. However, if you take vitamins from fresh natural sources every day you should get an adequate supply.

MINERALS

These occur in incredibly minute quantities in the body but are essential to many metabolic processes. They act like catalysts, affecting function although they are not actually used; when their work is done they are excreted in the urine and sweat, which means they must be replaced regularly from natural sources. It is not advisable to take capsule supplements of minerals as the dividing line between the required amount and an overdose is very fine and it is easy to disturb the entire mineral balance. Minerals are obtained mostly from herbs and vegetables, as plants extract minerals from the soil. Minerals help control the amount of water necessary to the life process; influence glandular performance; affect muscle responses; assist in nerve transmissions and help draw chemical substances in and out of cells. Scientists now consider that mineral balance is of the utmost importance and enables us to adjust to environmental pollution and stress. A balanced intake of fresh vegetables will provide an adequate amount of mineral elements.

WATER

Many people can survive for weeks without food, but not more than a few days without water. Our bodies are about two thirds water and the level remains remarkably constant. Water is lost through urine and sweat and it is replaced by the liquids we drink and by the water contained in all foods. It is healthy to drink at least a pint (three glasses) of water a day – in addition to water taken in tea or coffee or in soft drinks. There are four kinds of drinking water: hard, which contains calcium, magnesium and other salts; soft, containing sodium and often copper, iron and zinc; distilled water, which has had all minerals removed by a steam process; and mineral water, which is natural untreated water, with nothing added or removed – there are many varieties, some sparkling. Most municipal waters are purified with chlorine and some have fluorine too, but there is some controversy as to the value of this.

FOOD NUTRIENTS

A comprehensive balanced diet of fresh foods from all the food groups provides the necessary elements for body growth, repair and energy. This summary of the essential nutrients is a guide to function and source. Many foods provide energy and cell nourishment, as well as a combination of vitamins and minerals. The foods mentioned here are not the only sources of a particular element, but they are some of the best.

Nutrient	Function	Food
PROTEINS	The essential amino acids in proteins promote growth, build and repair body tissue, generally aid metabolism and provide energy	Meat, poultry, fish, milk, eggs, cheese, yogurt, nuts, seeds, whole cereals
CARBOHYDRATES Sugar	Gives quick energy	Fresh and dried fruits, honey, molasses
Starch	Source of heat and energy	Whole grains and cereals, whole-grain breads, tuber and root vegetables, peas, beans, lentils
Cellulose	Provides the bulk and fibre necessary for the digestive tract	Stalks, roots, bulbs, and fruits of vegetables
FATS	Stored in the body as reserve energy; insulate the body against heat loss; protect vital organs	Vegetable oils, fish oils, animal fats (minimum), milk, cheese, cream, nuts
VITAMINS Vitamin A (Retinol)	Helps repair body tissues and skeletal growth; promotes good eyesight; helps keep skin in good condition	Deep yellow foods such as apricots, butter, carrots, cheese, eggs, mangoes, papayas; liver, kidney; dark green vegetables like kale and broccoli, watercress, alfalfa sprouts
Vitamin B-1 (Thiamine)	Necessary for the conversion of carbohydrates into glucose for energy; important for nervous system, heart and liver	Poultry, lamb's liver, Brazil nuts, sunflower seeds, wheatgerm and wholewheat grains, rolled oats, brown rice
Vitamin B-2 (Riboflavin)	Helps to break down food for nutrition and energy; necessary for cell respiration and good vision	Milk, cheese, eggs, brewer's yeast, wheatgerm, wild rice, poultry, liver, kidney, almonds, avocado
Vitamin B-3 (Niacin)	Assists in the entire digestive process; important to mental health and the nervous system; most beneficial working in a team with the other B vitamins	Chicken, chicken liver, lamb's liver, kidneys, halibut, mackerel, sardines, peanuts, whole grains and bread

Nutrient	Function	Food
Vitamin B-5 (Pantothenic acid)	Involved in the metabolism of fatty acids; helps free energy from foods; essential for balanced functioning of the adrenal gland	Flesh foods, kidneys, lamb's liver, egg yolk, bran, brewer's yeast, whole grains, nuts
Vitamin B-6 (Pyridoxine)	Connected with growth and important in regulation of the nervous system; aids in metabolic breakdown of foods; helps form antibodies and red blood cells	Bananas, poultry, lamb's liver, mackerel, nuts, wheatgerm, whole grains and bread
Vitamin B-12 (Cyanocobalamin)	Essential for normal functioning of body cells, particularly those of bone marrow and the nervous system	Cheese, eggs, milk, poultry, fish, meat, liver, soy beans
Biotin (Vitamin B complex)	Helps to form fatty acids, burning them up with the carbohydrates for energy; necessary for healthy skin	Raw egg yolk, liver, kidney, black currants, molasses, rolled oats
Choline (Vitamin B complex)	Aids fat distribution from the liver; assists nerve transmission	Fish, heart, lentils, wheatgerm, whole grains, beans, lecithin granules
Folic acid (Vitamin B complex)	Helps form red blood cells and nucleic acids, essential for reproduction process	Liver, oysters, cabbage (raw), watercress, almonds, walnuts
Inositol (Vitamin B complex)	Together with choline, inositol forms lecithin, which keeps the liver free of fats	Bran, nuts, oats, sesame seeds, wheatgerm, lecithin granules
PABA (Vitamin B complex)	Enables other vitamin B elements to function properly	Broccoli, cabbage, kale, kidneys, liver, meat, poultry
Vitamin C (Ascorbic acid)	Maintains level of collagen necessary for the formation of connective tissue, bone, skin and cartilage; claimed to help some virus infections	Cabbage, cauliflower, broccoli, Brussels sprouts, green peppers, watercress, alfalfa sprouts, citrus fruits, black currants, strawberries
Vitamin D (Calciferol)	Essential for healthy teeth and bones as it helps take the calcium and phosphorus to the necessary building tissues	Exposure to sunshine, eggs, cod-liver-oil, halibut oil, mackerel, sardines, cheese
Vitamin E (Tocopherol)	Needed for normal metabolism, believed to improve circulatory system; used to increase fertility	Carrots, cabbage, cheese, eggs, olive oil, rolled oats, sunflower seeds, wheatgerm, wholewheat cereals and bread

Nutrient	Function	Food
Vitamin K	Prevents haemorrhaging and aids the normal blood-clotting process	Broccoli, cabbage, potatoes, eggs, oats, wheatgerm, wholewheat grains
MINERALS Calcium	Necessary to build and maintain bones and teeth; important for heart regulation and nerve transmission	Milk, cheese, almonds, olives, kelp and other seaweeds, sesame seeds, molasses, broccoli
Chlorine	In conjunction with sodium, is important in cell metabolism	Celery, lettuce, spinach, tomatoes, kelp, salt
Chromium	A trace mineral, helps regulate blood-sugar levels; believed to help keep the cholesterol level down	Bran, brewer's yeast, poultry, fruits, green vegetables, nuts
Cobalt	A trace mineral, necessary for function of vitamin B-12	Fruits, green vegetables, meat, whole-grain cereals
Copper	Significant in the production of red blood cells for the utilization of iron	Poultry, liver, kidney, shellfish, nuts, whole-grain cereals, lettuce, cabbage
Fluorine	Strengthens bones and teeth by helping to deposit calcium; counteracts tooth decay	Sea-food, fish, tea
Iodine	Important for the proper functioning of the thyroid gland	Shellfish, sea-food, sea salt, seaweeds, kelp
Iron	Very important mineral involved in oxidizing cells and forming haemoglobin	Offal – kidney, liver; shellfish, egg yolk, dark green, leafy vegetables, watercress, soy and sunflower seeds, whole-grain breads and cereals, molasses
Magnesium	Important in cell metabolism; necessary as a catalytic agent for other minerals and vitamins and for the nerve and muscle systems	Almonds, barley, molasses, nuts, sea-foods and sea-salt, olives, molasses
Manganese	Activates enzymes; influences blood-sugar levels and helps maintain reproductive processes; a trace mineral	Kidneys, parsley, watercress, spinach, cabbage, apricots, lentils, nuts, wheatgerm

Nutrient	Function	Food
Phosphorus	The most active of all minerals, important for growth and maintenance; together with calcium provides hard structure for bones; passes on genetic hereditary patterns	Meat, fish, eggs, cheese, wheatgerm, whole-grain cereals
Potassium	Often in partnership with sodium, maintaining a balance of fluids and important in muscle and nerve reactions	Sea-food, potatoes, green-leaf vegetables, soy beans, lima beans, bananas, apricots, figs
Selium	Not exactly known, but related to vitamin E in function; a trace mineral	Kidney, liver, nuts, sea-food, whole-grain cereals
Sodium	Works in combination with potassium and chloride; together they are often called electrolytes as they are significant in all cellular metabolism; protects the body against excess fluid loss	Poultry, green vegetables, kelp, sea salt, sea-food, water and wheatgerm
Sulphur	Helps in the formation of body tissue; necessary for activity of vitamins thiamine and biotin; a trace mineral	Milk, cheese, eggs, poultry, fish, beans, nuts, soy beans
Zinc	A trace mineral, influences the enzyme and protein pattern in digestion	Eggs, nuts, onions, shellfish, sunflower seeds, wheatgerm, bran

FOOD CATEGORIES

A daily eating plan should concentrate on fresh, wholesome food with as many raw items as possible. Thirty per cent of the total should comprise protein foods: dairy products, grains and wholewheat breads, nuts, seeds, legumes, fish, poultry and meat, but with much less emphasis on the meat sources. Sixty-five per cent of the diet should be vegetables and fruits, particularly vegetables – leafy varieties, salads, roots, tubers, stalks, fruits; in the fruit category, balance is needed between citrus, orchard, berry and tropical fruits. Five per cent should be of fat origin, but use the vegetable oils, nuts and margarine rather than butter. The main food categories are as follows.

DAIRY PRODUCTS

Milk: One of the most valuable foods, for a single pint (6 dl.) contains about a fifth of the daily nutrient requirement. Naturopathic doctors, however, are against excessive intake of milk – more milk does not necessarily mean more benefit, particularly in adults; one or two glasses a day is sufficient, less if there are certain disease complications. The quality of milk varies according to the breed of cow, climate, fodder and season. At its best, a pint a day will provide 25 per cent of protein needs, including an almost complete set of amino acids, a maximum amount of calcium, 50 per cent of riboflavin, 30 per cent of vitamin A and a little more than 15 per cent of thiamine. The most nutritional benefits from milk are obtained from untreated milk, which has to come from specially licensed farms and dairies. In western countries there are strict rules about natural milk production because of the possibility of brucellosis (undulant fever), which is passed on to humans if the milk is not heat-treated. Normally the heating process of pasteurization destroys milk-borne bacteria; this process has little effect on the nutritional value of milk and is a significant health safeguard. *Homogenized milk* is treated so that the fat globules are evenly distributed throughout. For *skimmed milk* the fat is removed; the fat-soluble vitamins such as A and D are lost but the protein, carbohydrate and vitamin C values remain intact. Milk contains a fair amount of invisible fat and some water. *Dried milk* preserves the proteins and the vitamins are only slightly reduced in quantity and quality.

Yogurt: Contains more protein and riboflavin than milk, and, although there is scepticism about its claims of rejuvenation and prolonging life, there is no doubt that it is a valuable contentrated nutrient.

Cheese: Richer in protein than meat, fish or poultry because its basis is the concentrated protein of milk – the part that forms the curd. It is a good source of vitamins A, D, E and B-2, rich in phosphorus and calcium. Unfortunately it can be high in fat and cholesterol. Cottage cheese and other skimmed milk cheeses are nourishing and lack the fat content; harder cheeses contain less fat than soft ones. Cow's milk is the most common in cheese-making, but sometimes goat's milk and occasionally ewe's milk are also used. Variations in flavour depend on fodder, water and the area, also the method of making and maturing the cheese – some cheeses ripen in a few days while others take several years.

Eggs: Not strictly a dairy product, but they usually come under this category. No other food contains so many nutrients. Eggs are particularly high in protein of excellent quality, with most of the required amino acids present. They provide calcium and iron and are a fine source of vitamins A, B-2 and D. The only drawback is that eggs contain a fair amount of fat – about 12 per cent, with almost all of it in the yolk. For this reason many nutritionists recommend only one egg a day, some only three a week. Brown and white eggs are equally nutritious, and though great stress is often put on the special merits of the free-range egg, there is not much difference nutritionally between it and the battery egg. Differences in diet cause variations in the colour of the yolk from pale yellow to orange. Eggs will stay fresh at room temperature for two weeks, in the refrigerator for three. As well as hens' eggs there are turkey, goose and duck eggs, though the latter contain more fat; also quail and plover eggs.

GRAINS

A staple food, plentiful and nutritious; an inexpensive and important source of energy, containing some protein and fat, with an assortment of vitamins and minerals. Grains are eaten as cereals or ground into flour. Because of their high starch content, they have the reputation of being fattening, but this is not necessarily so.

Wheat: The most valuable of grains with two main varieties, one for use in flour and bread-making, the other as the basis of pasta. Wheat contains more protein than any other cereal, and the amount of other nutrients depends on the degree of milling: after the outer coat of the wheat is extracted, the grain goes through a series of grinding and sifting operations. The fineness of the sieve determines the extraction rate. If nothing is sieved out, the flour is wholewheat. The 'rougher' the flour, the more nutritious the bread, as it contains more protein, fat and iron, and the vitamins B-1, B-2, B-3. The final sifting will produce the whitest flour with virtually no nutrients left. Gluten, a combination of two proteins, becomes viscous when water is added and so produces a dough. The dough rises by means of gaseous bubbles of carbon dioxide given off by fermenting yeast. Pasta is made from semolina, which is the ground endosperm (inner layer) of a special variety of wheat.

Rye: The protein value is lower than that of wheat; it contains a little less fat but the same proportion of vitamins and minerals. It has a lower gluten content than wheat, so bread made with rye is dense in texture. The variations in colour depend on the extraction rate in milling – the darkest is pumpernickel.

Oats: Very rich in protein and a fine source of the B vitamins; the protein level is not as high as that of wheat and it has a little more fat content. Oatmeal lacks gluten and so cannot be made into bread, but porridge is one of the most nutritious breakfast foods. Raw rolled oats are the basis of Bircher muesli, recommended in almost every nature clinic.

Corn: Has a lower protein level than wheat and does not contain a complete set of amino acids; it has a high fat content and provides vitamins in the B group. It does not have enough gluten to make bread; it is coarsely ground into cornmeal and made into the Italian staple, polenta, among other dishes; when pulverized it becomes cornstarch. One of its more important products is corn oil, a good polyunsaturated fat.

Barley: Contains some protein, but less than wheat; a good source of B vitamins, especially B-3. It has a low fat content. Pot barley is the most nutritious as it is the whole grain with only the outer husk removed; pearl barley is more refined, lacking the bran and germ as well as the husk.

Rice: Lower in protein than wheat, but otherwise nutritionally similar, with a slightly lower fat level. Brown rice is the healthiest, the husk only being taken away, leaving the protein, fat, minerals and vitamin B elements. Short-grain and long-grain white rice have a higher starch content because the bran and germ are also removed during milling and polishing; white rice loses 2 per cent of its protein, almost all of its fat and minerals and, worst of all, its vitamin B-1, which is completely destroyed. Lack of vitamin B-1 causes beriberi, and is a real danger in countries where rice is the staple diet. A process called parboiling minimizes the loss and produces rice that is not so white, but more nutritious.

MEAT

Beef, veal, lamb and pork are all high-quality proteins and, in particular, give a well-balanced group of amino acids. They are rich in the B vitamins, especially B-1, B-3 and B-12. Iron, phosphorus, potassium, sodium and magnesium are present in appreciable amounts. Meat is digested slowly, thus satisfying hunger for some time and providing delayed energy. Unfortunately, meat often contains a high proportion of saturated fat as well as a moderate amount of cholesterol: pork is the worst in this respect. Fat is not only on the outer surface of meats, but is marbled within the flesh and fibres as well; the percentage of such fat is higher in cattle specially reared and fed for quick growth and human consumption than in free-grazing herds. Offal is reputed to be specially nutritious. To some extent this is true, as it contains less fat than the flesh meats, is equal in protein value and higher in iron, vitamin A, B-1 and B-2; unfortunately it contains twice the amount of cholesterol. Bacon, which is salted and smoked pork, has the same protein and energy value as pork, but some of the vitamins B-1 and B-3 are lost in the salting, while the saltiness itself is bad for certain metabolisms and diseases. Wild game such as hare, deer, boar and bear all have relatively lean meat.

POULTRY

Chicken is high in protein and low in fat, a good source of the B vitamins and iron. It contains some cholesterol, but not as much as meat. Free-range chickens are superior to those produced on battery farms, not only in taste but in health-giving qualities. Chickens freeze well and retain their value. Turkey is similar in nutrients to chicken – high in protein, low in fat. Ducks and geese have almost twice as much saturated fat as chicken and turkey, though the other constituents remain the same. Wild birds – partridge, pheasant, guinea hen and so on – have leaner meat with a good protein content.

FISH

When fresh, fish is one of the most valuable foods; the protein content can be from 15 – 20 per cent and it contains most of the important amino acids. As a source of protein it is superior to meat because the fat is polyunsaturated; it varies in quantity according to the time of year as well as the type of fish. Oily fish contains more fat than white fish, but because of its nature this is of little importance as regards health. Fish contains less cholesterol than meat and provides a balanced supply of the B vitamins; oily fish, however, contains vitamin D and vitamin B-3, which is absent in white fish. The value of fish relies upon it being fresh – it quickly putrifies. However, freezing the fish on the trawlers keeps it 'fresh' for up to three months, but it must be cooked as soon as it is defrosted.

Shellfish are high in protein and vitamins B-2 and B-3; they provide significant amounts of iron and calcium. Shellfish are low in fat, but contain twice as much cholesterol as other fish. Lobster has more cholesterol than meat and oysters more still.

NUTS

Extremely high in protein and energy; some nuts have as high a percentage of protein as meat, with the added bonus that their fat is of vegetable origin and therefore polyunsaturated and not detrimental to health. They contain the B vitamins and a wide range of minerals, iron being the most prevalent. They are a highly concentrated source of energy and nutrients. The nutritional value varies; for protein value pine nuts and peanuts are best, then almonds, cashews and Brazils. Pistachios are unusually rich in iron.

VEGETABLES

Green Vegetables

The darker green the leaves the more chlorophyll they contain, and this is related to the amount of carotene, which can be converted into vitamin A in the body. All green vegetables are high in vitamins and minerals, providing almost all the necessary elements. Spinach, broccoli tops, kale, cabbage, cauliflower and brussels sprouts are all valuable sources of vitamin C, but because it dissolves in water, the percentage can fall by half on cooking. Many green vegetables can be easily and pleasantly eaten raw, and are then at their most nutritious. They make a most important contribution to health and one or other of them should be taken daily. As well as being lost in cooking, some vitamins are diminished even on exposure to air, so leave preparation until the last minute and never allow vegetables to soak for long in cold water – a quick rinse is enough to get rid of dirt and any insecticide film. Cook vegetables quickly and eat immediately; never use bicarbonate of soda in the water to retain the green as this kills the vitamin C; use lemon juice instead. Celery, bamboo and fennel are not very high in vitamin and mineral content, but are an excellent source of necessary fibre. Asparagus has a considerable amount of protein and is rich in folic acid.

Salad Leaves

Mostly water and bulk, requiring a fair amount of chewing – all of which makes them valuable foods. Most leaves are rich in vitamin C, the greener ones being the best. Wild salad leaves such as dandelion have the most nutrients. Watercress is one of the best, being high in carotene (for vitamin

A), vitamin C and iron. The most beneficial salad leaves are sprouts from seeds, which can be grown in a few days. Alfalfa can be grown in a jar with water and takes from three to six days to sprout; it is high in vitamins A, B-complex, C, D, E and K, together with useful amounts of calcium, iron, phosphorus and the trace minerals, and a significant protein content.

Legumes and Pulses

Peas and beans provide more energy and protein than any green or root vegetable; they are also a good source of B vitamins and some vitamin C. All varieties of green beans contain much more vitamin C – twice as much eaten raw as when cooked. The amount of protein in the seeds of legumes varies; runner beans have only 1 per cent but soy beans have 30 per cent; kidney beans have a higher protein content than meat. All can be eaten in quantity without any fear of fat.

Dried seeds from the pods are called pulses and in theory are as rich in protein as meat, and also contain iron and a large amount of vitamin B elements. However, because they have to be soaked in water before cooking protein and energy ingredients are lost. Nevertheless, it is a good idea to increase the ratio of pulses in the diet – haricot beans, broad beans, lima beans, kidney beans, black-eyed beans, chick peas, lentils and soy beans.

Vegetable Fruits

Most have little nutritional merit, but they are non-fattening, being on average about 90 per cent water with only a trace of fat and little carbohydrate. Their fibrous bulk satisfies hunger and, because of the considerable chewing necessary, induces production of saliva and gastric juices. In addition, they aid the more nutritious foods to pass through the digestive tract. Herbalists value the powers of many vegetable fruits, particularly the cucumber. Eaten raw, the tomato is a good source of carotene and vitamin C. Sweet peppers are rich in vitamin C.

Tubers, Roots and Bulbs

Potatoes are less fattening than bread, but contain a useful amount of starch for energy; they are a valuable source of vitamin C and vitamins B-1 and B-3. They also contain a substantial amount of protein, but this is highly concentrated just below the skin – if you peel a potato up to a quarter of its protein is lost. It is better to bake or boil potatoes unpeeled. The vitamin C can be lost in too much water or too much boiling. Sweet potatoes are useful for the carotene and vitamin C content. Roots are starchy but low in calories and at their highest nutrient level in spring and summer. Minerals are available in beets, turnips, rutabagas and parsnips. Again do not scrape or peel these root vegetables, otherwise much of the value is lost. Horse-radish is exceptionally high in vitamin C; kohlrabi contains as much vitamin C as oranges. Of all the root vegetables carrots are the most useful, being a major source of carotene, which is converted into vitamin A. The onion family – including leeks, chives, garlic, shallots – are high in sulphur and low in calories but nutritionists say that they are of little nutritional value. Herbalists and naturopaths think highly of their healing powers, however (see pages 113–14).

Fungi

Many wild mushrooms have useful amounts of vitamin D, and both wild and cultivated varieties are good sources of vitamin B-3, potassium and phosphorus. Mushrooms are used mostly for flavour; they are most beneficial when added raw to salads. Check the identification of any wild fungi, as many are poisonous.

SEAWEEDS

Particularly rich in minerals, especially calcium, potassium, sodium and iodine. Seaweed could provide an interesting addition to our diet. It can be eaten as a vegetable, fried or boiled; the most common varieties in use are bladder wrack and knotted wrack, which can also be used as flavourings for fish dishes. A brown seaweed known as kelp is made into a salt or seasoning.

FRUITS

All fruits provide natural sugar, and therefore energy, without the harmful effects of refined and processed sugars. They also quench thirst, as most fruits have a high water content; in addition they are a good source of fibre. Orchard fruits such as apples and pears have minerals and vitamin C. The more succulent orchard fruits like peaches, plums and apricots contain more vitamins and minerals; in particular, the nectarine, with vitamin C, carotene (for vitamin A production) and vitamin B-2. Apricots are a very good source of potassium and magnesium – indeed they are considered as being responsible for longevity in certain parts of the world. The citrus fruits are valued for their vitamin C, though there are richer sources in the vegetable world. It is important to eat an orange at the right time for maximum benefit; the riper it is the less vitamin C it contains. The vine fruits – grapes and melons – are mostly water, but they are full of minerals, particularly potassium. Berries are interesting as, despite their very high water content – 90 per cent on average – they are rich in minerals such as calcium and in the vitamins B-1 and B-2; they also contain carotene for the production of vitamin A and they are a particularly good source of vitamin C – black currants have four times as much as citrus fruits. Tropical fruits are high in carbohydrates; bananas also have a fair amount of vitamin C, carotene and vitamin B-2; guavas are very high in vitamin C and so is pineapple, but the vitamin is lost in canning.

Dried Fruits

These are good sources of energy, their carbohydrate content being relatively high, and they also contain some protein, vitamins and minerals. Figs are high in fibre as well as in the B vitamins and minerals, particularly iron. Dried apricots are a good source of vitamin C and contain more protein than any other dried fruit. Currants and raisins have a fairly high content of iron. Dates never really dry out, but because two thirds of the content is sugar they should be eaten in moderation, even though they are rich in minerals, especially iron.

HEALTH HERBS IN COOKING: GUIDE TO GENERAL USE

In cooking, herbs are not eaten in sufficient quantity to be significant medicinally, though they do contain valuable vitamins and minerals. Their most important contribution is their distinctive flavour; in addition they often help counterbalance any adverse properties of a particular food.

This is a basic guide and by no means rigid; experiment with various combinations, using small quantities to begin with.

ANGELICA

Slightly liquorice-flavoured plant. Leaves are candied for a dessert decoration and the seeds can be added to pastry. The oil distilled from the seeds and roots is used for flavouring wines and liqueurs and gives an unusual taste to sweet sauces.

ANISEED

A subtle liquorice flavour, widely used in baking cakes, biscuits, bread rolls and pastry for fruit pies. It is grown mainly for its seeds, though the leaves can be eaten in salads and as garnishes. To release the full flavour of the seeds, crush them between greaseproof paper with a rolling pin.

BASIL

Particularly good with fish, egg and tomato dishes, and useful in all savoury dishes including those with cheese. Gives flavour to potato and rice salads, soups and stews. The chopped fresh herb goes well with pasta.

BAY

Use it in moderation, fresh or dry, for stuffings, stocks, sauces, court bouillon, marinades, casseroles, vegetable cooking. It is recommended with corned beef and tongue and gives a subtle flavour when boiled with artichokes, eggplant or potatoes. Bay leaves dry well and hold their aromatic qualities for years.

BORAGE

Only good when fresh, as all the flavour disappears in drying. The leaves impart a cucumber taste in juices, fish sauces or white aspics. Traditional in fruit punches and summer drinks, and as a garnish. Young borage can be cooked like spinach or served in salads.

BOUQUET GARNI

A standard combination of herbs used in soups, stews and casseroles: 2 sprigs of parsley, 2 sprigs of chervil, 1 sprig of marjoram, 1 sprig of thyme, $\frac{1}{2}$ bay leaf. Put in a firmly tied muslin bag.

CARAWAY

The leaves can be used sparingly in soups and stews. The seeds are used in making breads, particularly rye, and give seed cake its name. The oil is the basic flavouring of the liqueur kummel. Overcooking makes the seeds bitter, so for soups and stews wrap them in a cloth and add only for the final 30 minutes of cooking. For salads and when cooked with vegetables – they are particularly good with cabbage – release the flavour by crushing the seeds first. The roots can be boiled and eaten like carrots.

CHERVIL

One of the 'bouquet garni' mixture. It is similar in appearance to parsley, though more delicate and ferny; the leaves are spicy, tasting slightly of aniseed. It enhances veal and chicken dishes, omelettes and salads. Essential as a garnish and for bearnaise and vinaigrette sauce. Garnish soups with the chopped leaves.

CHIVES

Used whenever a mild onion flavour is needed. They can be folded into cream cheese, egg dishes, mashed potatoes and cooked rice or omelettes. A sprinkling of chopped chives greatly improves salads and raw vegetables. Excellent in green sauce with boiled beef and as a garnish with new potatoes, fish and hors d'oeuvres. The aroma of chives is destroyed by long cooking so add the leaves either fresh or dried, at the final moment.

CORIANDER

The seeds have a very spicy taste and are used in breads and cakes. They are excellent for pickles and the subtle aroma gives an interesting undertone to soups and casseroles. It is also important in curry powder blends.

CUMIN

Very aromatic seeds, used in the making of curry, chilli powder and chutney. It is baked in unleavened bread, such as rye, and used to enliven bean and rice dishes.

DILL

Both seeds and leaves are used in sour cream, fish, bean, cucumber and cabbage dishes, as well as in potato salad and with new potatoes. Dill seed is sprinkled on breads, rolls and fruit pies. It is also used in pickling cucumbers, and bland vegetables are greatly improved by its flavour. The finely chopped leaves are good in creamed potatoes, white sauces, cottage or cream cheeses.

FENNEL

The leaves and seeds are used like dill, especially with fat fish (bass, mackerel, etc.), with beans, lentils, rice and potatoes. The seeds go into breads and cakes, on top of rolls and fruit tarts and in cheese mixtures and spreads. Fennel gives an aromatic taste to fish and meat dishes, especially pork, liver and kidneys.

GARLIC

One of the most versatile of culinary herbs, it provides a special penetrating flavour and actually helps digestion. It can be overpowering at first, so begin with small quantities, increasing gradually. Cloves of garlic can go into soups, meat or vegetables, casseroles; it is good with roast lamb and pungent with bread. Important in salad dressings – rub salad bowl with a cut, peeled, garlic clove or add a crushed clove to the dressing,

allow to stand for an hour to infuse the flavour. Remove the garlic before using the dressing.

LOVAGE

The leaves can be used as a celery substitute with stews or tongue; stems may be blanched and eaten like celery, or candied like angelica. It has a strong yeast-like flavour and acts as a substitute for meat and bones in soups and casseroles.

MARJORAM

Its wild form is called oregano and is stronger in flavour, particularly when dried. Both are zesty, good in potato and dumpling dishes, with pasta and rice, in stuffings and forcemeats of all kinds. It is rubbed into lamb, mutton and pork before roasting and is used as a flavouring in vinegar and wine brews. Together with thyme and sage, it comprises the traditional mixed herbs: 1 part each of marjoram and thyme to 2 parts sage.

MUSTARD

Culinary mustards come from the ripe seeds and in powder form can make a subtle, tangy, difference to cheese dishes, salad dressing, white sauce, mayonnaise and cabbage, and in the cooking of salted meats. Classically served with cold meats; also used in pickles and chutney.

PARSLEY

This common garden herb is a prime health giver as well as a most versatile culinary herb. It can be used with practically every dish. Because its flavour is fresh and not dominant, it can go with other herbs in many dishes, especially as a garnish,

where its visual appeal and health value are plus factors. It helps salads, soups, stews and stuffings; it goes into sauces, fish and egg dishes.

ROSEMARY

The leaves are very pungent and should be used cautiously in cooking. Important in marinades for lamb, rabbit, veal and pork. Gives spice to stuffings.

SAGE

One of the best herbs to counteract the richness of foods such as fatty meats, pork, sausages, duck, goose and oily fish; it also combines well with bean and pea soups and with cheese and onion combinations; much used in stuffings.

SORREL

The leaves have a fresh, slightly acid taste, good in soups and sauces and as an accompaniment to egg dishes and cold meat. Combines well with other herbs or leaves, especially lettuce – a French dressing sweetened with honey balances the acidity.

TARRAGON

A spicy, aromatic herb imparting an interesting taste to bland food such as fish, eggs, soups, poultry, liver and sweetbreads. The leaves are used in sauces, marinades, salads and stuffings. Essential in bearnaise and hollandaise sauces.

THYME

Use in moderation in hearty dishes such as mutton, pork, shellfish and chicken, and in stuffings; best combined with vegetables in main dishes.

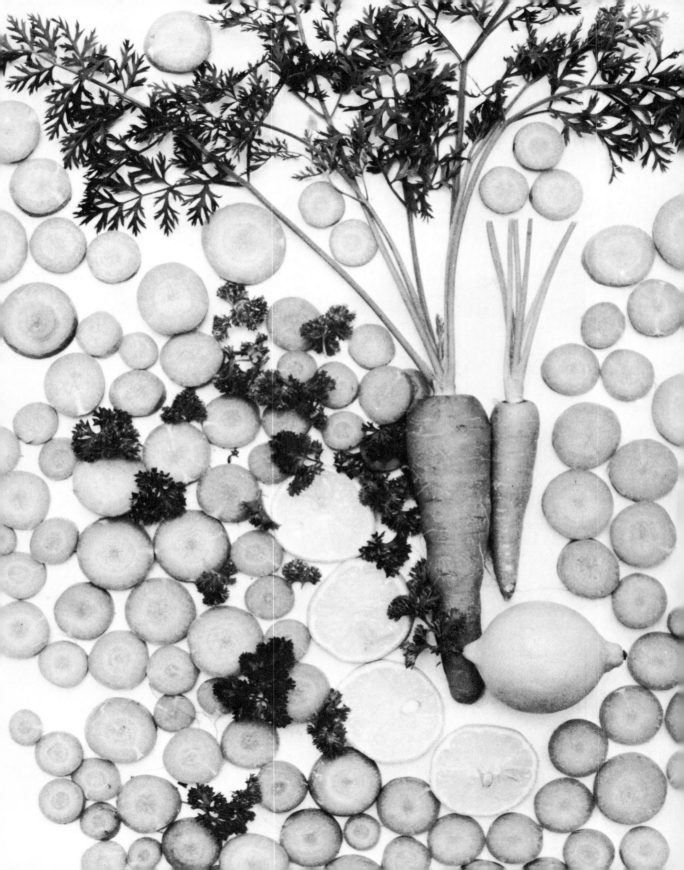

2

COOKING

Until recently one of the complaints against health food and dietary régimes was that the recipes were uninspired and resulted in dishes that looked and were unappetizing. Now, thanks to a French master chef, the whole philosophy has changed and we have the means of making splendid dishes that conform to the principles of healthy eating.

The new approach originated with Michel Guérard, who calls his technique *cuisine minceur* (slimming cooking). He experimented with the traditional recipes and methods of French cooking and evolved alternative ways to retain the high standard with the minimum use of fats, eggs, cream, butter, starches and sugar. The result is delicious delicate food that is perfect for the palate and the body. His book *Cuisine Minceur* (available in an English translation by Caroline Conran) gives a detailed account of his methods and recipes. He runs a spa restaurant, La Maison des Prés et des Sources d'Eugénie, at Eugénie-les-Bains in south-west France.

Many of his dishes are for experienced cooks and those with time but the principles of *cuisine minceur* can be applied to everyday cooking, keeping time and ingredients down to a minimum, and still producing attractive flavourings and sauces.

One of the basic rules is to use the freshest ingredients. Butter, fats, creams, eggs, flours and sugar are used only in minimum amounts. Sauces can often be thickened with puréed vegetables or non-fat cheeses, or may be simply reduced stock.

As much fat as possible must be trimmed away from meat. When fat – a little butter or vegetable oil – is used for browning meat, remove from the sautéing pan and wipe dry before doing the rest of the cooking. Adding a little white wine or lemon juice to sautéed vegetables will counteract the fat.

Cooking time for all dishes is short, particularly for vegetables, which should preferably be steamed. When on a diet portions should naturally be limited, and M. Guérard stresses that there must be only two or three courses for lunch and three for dinner. Equipment is very important for this type of cooking; heavy pans and casseroles mean that food can be cooked quickly at a high temperature without burning. In this way flavour and food value are retained. Steamers and poachers are necessary; an electric blender or food processor is essential, as puréeing, blending and liquidizing are much used. The following are a combination of *cuisine minceur* and the basic rules of healthy cooking.

COOKING METHODS

ROASTING

The meat or poultry can be browned first in a little oil or butter on top of the stove; excess fat must be wiped off before the meat is put in a roasting pan with herbs and flavourings. It can be covered with foil to prevent drying out or burning – the foil should be removed for the last few minutes to crisp the top. A chicken can retain fat under the skin, so this should be released by pricking with a fine needle just before serving.

BRAISING

Again the food is browned first on top of the stove, wiped clean of fat and cooked in a casserole in stock. Any remaining fat can be skimmed off the sauce at the last moment.

FOIL COOKING

Meat, fish and poultry can be completely wrapped in foil. This method has the advantage that no additional fat or oil is added, and the food cooks in its own juices, with any added flavourings.

SAUTÉING

A heavy skillet is essential, as sautéing should be done in very little oil or butter over a high flame. Meat or poultry should have any extra fat wiped away; vegetables can have wine or lemon juice added. If ingredients are to be returned to the skillet for further cooking wipe the pan dry too.

STEAMING

The food is cooked entirely by the steam from boiling water below. The food should be placed on a perforated rack over the liquid and the pan then covered. In *cuisine minceur* stock is often used instead of water to give more flavour.

POACHING

The food is completely immersed in boiling water or stock; a medium heat is needed for the best results. Often fat is released, but this can be skimmed off both during and at the end of cooking.

STOCKS

These are the mainstay of slim and healthy cooking; they are used for poaching, steaming and braising, and at times to pour over a roast. They are the basis of sauces, soups and gravies. A supply of home-made stock should always be on hand. It is easy to make – although it takes a long time to cook – and can be stored in the refrigerator. Three basic stocks are beef, chicken and fish; any fat should be skimmed off as it comes to the surface during cooking.

Beef Stock
2 lb. (1 kg.) beef bones
   and pieces
1 veal knuckle and bones
3 carrots
3 onions
2 stalks celery
2 tomatoes
20 cups cold water
1 cup dry white wine
1 bouquet garni
freshly ground pepper
a little sea-salt

Brown the meat bones and pieces in a heavy deep pan, without fat. Chop up the vegetables and add them; pour in the water, wine and seasonings. Bring to the boil; reduce the heat and simmer for a minimum of 3 hours, skimming off fat as it appears. Strain, cool, cover and refrigerate. If more fat appears on the surface remove before use.

Chicken Stock
Chicken stock is made in exactly the same way, but replace the beef with 4 lb. (2 kg.) chicken carcasses, wings, necks and other small pieces.

Fish Stock
2 lb. (1 kg.) fish bones and heads
2 sliced onions
2 stalks celery
2 tablespoons chopped parsley
1 bay leaf
½ teaspoon thyme or tarragon
20 cups water
1 cup dry white wine
pinch of salt
freshly ground pepper

Put all ingredients in a deep pan, bring to the boil, reduce the heat and simmer for about 1 hour. Strain, cool, refrigerate.

MARINADES

These give a good flavour; wines, vinegars or lemon juice, together with a selection of herbs, can be used. The longer the food is marinated the more flavour it will have.

SAUCES

Equal amounts of butter and flour – as little as possible – are the basis of a roux to which can be added vegetable purées, an egg yolk, skimmed cheese, dried milk with water, yogurt or stock.

On the following pages are recipes which, to a large extent, use *cuisine minceur* principles but also embrace wholefood ideas; some are for extra nourishment rather than slimming. Breads have been included, as it is healthy to make your own. The entire approach is one of simplicity and care. None of the recipes takes long to make; many are suitable for entertaining as well as everyday use.

Give some thought to the menu; try to get away from the standard three courses, the main one being meat and two vegetables. Think more about soup, which can be a meal in itself; experiment with grains for main courses, salads for appetizers. For dessert, fruit is the answer, preferably fresh, or prepared in such a way as to preserve vitamins and give extra flavour.

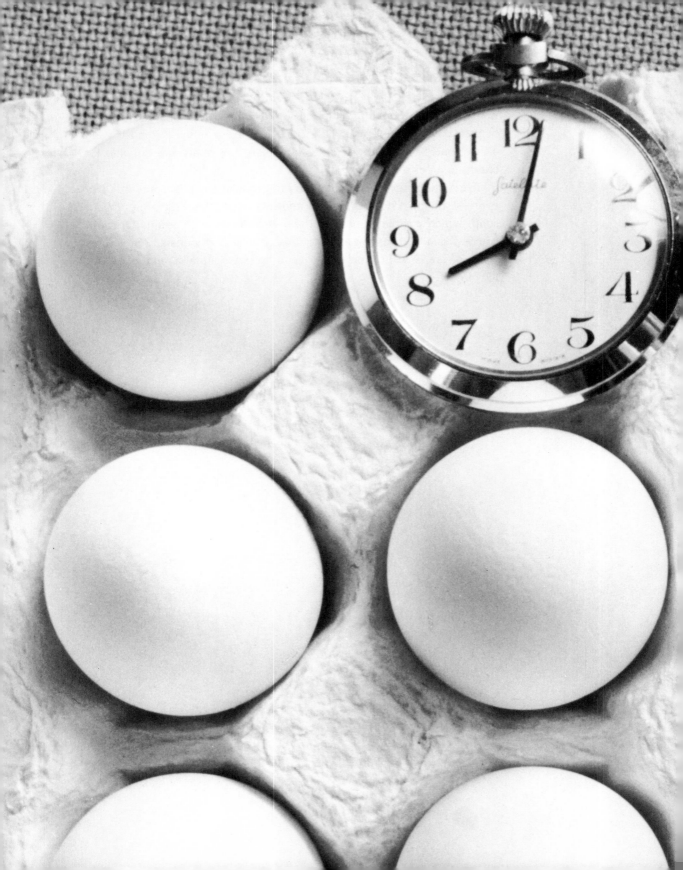

3

RECIPES

SAUCES

Horse-radish Sauce

½ cup cream

2 teaspoons cider vinegar

1 teaspoon mustard powder

½ teaspoon salt

1 teaspoon raw sugar

2 tablespoons freshly grated
   horse-radish

Whip the cream and stir in the vinegar, mustard, salt, sugar and, finally, the horse-radish. Leave for at least 30 minutes before use.

Fennel Sauce

½ cup fennel leaves

½ cup mint leaves

½ cup parsley leaves

¼ lb. butter, melted

Wash the herbs well, put them in a pan and cover with water; boil until soft, 6 – 8 minutes; drain and dry, then chop finely. Add the melted butter and serve right away. Particularly good with fish.

Cold Mustard Sauce

2 hard-boiled eggs

2 teaspoons grated onion

1 tablespoon prepared mustard

1 teaspoon sugar

1 – 2 tablespoons olive oil

2 tablespoons cider vinegar

1 tablespoon cream

Chop the eggs finely and mix with the rest of the ingredients. Good with boiled or cold meat and fish dishes.

Apple and Elderberry Sauce

2 apples

2 sprays elderberries

3 tablespoons water

1 tablespoon raw sugar

Peel, core and slice the apples and put in a pan together with the elderberries (pulled from stalks, fresh or dried); add the water and sugar, simmer slowly until the apples are soft, stirring often. Serve hot or cold.

Horse-radish Bread Sauce

¼ cup grated fresh horse-radish
3 tablespoons breadcrumbs
1½ cups milk
1 tablespoon butter or margarine
1 teaspoon lemon juice
salt to taste

Soak the breadcrumbs and horse-radish in the milk for 20 minutes, then slowly bring to simmering point. Take off the heat, stir in the butter, lemon juice and salt. Cover and allow to stand in a warm place until serving. Goes well with turkey, duck, goose or roast beef.

Basic Tomato Purée

1 garlic clove
a little olive oil
10 ripe tomatoes (or a can of Italian
    plum tomatoes)
salt and pepper
a bunch of basil

Put a little olive oil in a deep pan; finely chop the garlic and brown slightly; add the tomatoes and salt and pepper to taste; cover the pan and stew very slowly until the tomatoes are a pulp; it is not necessary to add water. Pass through a fine sieve to remove seeds and skins. Put in jars with a leaf of basil and cover with a film of olive oil. Keep in the refrigerator. This is a basic sauce for pasta dishes, rice and soups, to which any dried herbs may be added for flavouring.

Green Sauce

1 clove of garlic
3 or 4 sprigs of parsley
½ oz. (15 g.) capers
1 anchovy
3 pitted olives
1 hard-boiled egg yolk
1 heaped tablespoon bread soaked
    in 1 tablespoon vinegar
1¼ cups olive oil
salt and pepper

Chop the garlic and parsley very finely and put in the blender with the capers, anchovy, olives, egg yolk and bread. When finely ground, gradually add the oil and finally the vinegar; season with salt and pepper. Eat with boiled meats and poultry.

Sage and Onion Sauce

1 oz. (30 g.) finely chopped onion
½ oz. (15 g.) finely chopped sage
    leaves
8 teaspoons water
salt and pepper
1 oz. (30 g.) breadcrumbs
½ cup stock, gravy or melted
    butter

Put the onion and sage in a pan with the water and simmer slowly for 10 minutes; season with salt and pepper, add the breadcrumbs and mix well; then pour in the broth, gravy or melted butter and simmer a little longer.

Sorrel Purée

2 lb. (1 kg.) sorrel
2 tablespoons margarine
1¼ cups cream
3 eggs
salt and freshly ground pepper

Clean and wash the sorrel, cook for 6 – 8 minutes in a little lightly salted water, drain and chop finely. Put the margarine in a skillet and sauté the sorrel in it for a few minutes; add the cream and the 3 eggs, previously beaten; stir constantly with a wooden spoon until the mixture thickens; season with pepper to taste. It is good as a garnish for hearty meat dishes, particularly pork. It can also be quickly converted into a soup by adding stock.

Spanish Sauce

3 cloves garlic
½ cup olive oil
½ cup sifted plain flour
5 cups stock
2 tablespoons chopped parsley
salt and pepper
½ cup cooked peas
5 cooked asparagus tips, chopped

Chop the garlic cloves and brown in the oil. When the garlic is just beginning to colour stir in the flour and gradually add the hot stock and then the chopped parsley; season with salt and pepper. Simmer the sauce, stirring constantly, until it is reduced by half. Add the peas and asparagus tips and simmer for 10 minutes longer. This sauce can be poured over boiled eggs and fish, or used as a garnish for potatoes and bland vegetables.

Cucumber Sauce

1 cucumber
12 seedless grapes
small bunch parsley
1 carton sour cream or yogurt
pinch of ground chilli
salt and pepper

Peel and dice the cucumber, sprinkle with salt and allow to drain. (The salt takes away the excess water in the cucumber.) Slice the grapes and finely chop the parsley. Fold into the sour cream, add the chilli and season to taste. Chill and serve cold.

Aïoli

12 cloves garlic
3 egg yolks
1½ cups olive oil
1 teaspoon lemon juice
salt to taste

Peel and mash the garlic cloves with a little salt; put in a bowl and stir in the egg yolks one by one; when blended, beat in the oil slowly, starting in drops; finally add the lemon juice.

Mixed Herbs and Breadcrumb Seasoning
1 tablespoon butter or margarine
1 cup soft wholewheat breadcrumbs
1 tablespoon finely chopped white onion
1 teaspoon dried sage
½ teaspoon dried thyme
½ teaspoon dried marjoram
a pinch of salt and pepper
1 teaspoon lemon juice
1 egg yolk

Cut the butter into small pieces and mix all the ingredients together well, binding finally with the yolk of an egg. An unusual tang is given if a pinch of curry powder is also added. Use to stuff poultry or boned meat.

SOUPS

French Garlic Soup
24 cloves garlic
2 tablespoons butter
1 tablespoon olive oil
7½ cups hot stock (vegetable, beef or chicken)
salt and pepper
pinch allspice
3 egg yolks
3 tablespoons olive oil
croutons

Peel and chop the garlic, brown slowly in the butter and oil. Pour over the hot stock; season with salt, freshly ground pepper and a pinch of allspice. Simmer for 15 minutes; strain. Return to a low heat. Beat the yolks with the olive oil, add a little warm stock, mix well and add to the pan. Stir until the mixture is thoroughly blended, but do not allow to boil. Serve with croutons; garnish with parsley – an optional extra.

Garbure
4 potatoes
4 carrots
1 large cabbage – as green as possible
½ lb. (250 g.) cooked white beans
1 ham bone or ¼ lb. (125 g.) bacon
1 bouquet garni
6¼ cups water
salt and black pepper

Chop the potatoes and carrots, shred the cabbage and put them in a pan with the white beans, ham bone or bacon and the bouquet garni. Pour over the water and bring to the boil; simmer for 40 minutes in a covered pan; remove the bouquet garni and add salt and freshly ground pepper to taste. Remove the meat or bacon. Chop meat into small pieces and return to soup; or cut the rind off the bacon and chop the remainder.

Carrot and Thyme Soup

1 lb. (½ kg.) chopped carrots
1 chopped onion
½ lb. (250 g.) tomatoes, peeled and chopped
1 clove garlic, chopped
8 branches fresh thyme or 2 teaspoons dried thyme
7½ cups stock
salt and pepper
juice of 1 lemon or orange

Put all the ingredients except the fruit juice in a pan. Simmer over low heat, seasoning to taste during cooking, until the carrots are cooked. Remove the twigs of thyme; put soup through a blender; at the last moment before serving stir in the orange or lemon juice; the soup looks decorative garnished with parsley.

Borage Soup

1 lb. (½ kg.) potatoes
½ cup borage leaves
3¾ cups milk
salt and pepper
2 teaspoons fresh cream or yogurt

Peel and cut potatoes, cook in lightly salted water until soft, drain and mash. Chop the borage leaves finely. Add the milk to the mashed potatoes, stirring well until blended. Put the pan on low heat, add the borage, salt and pepper to taste; simmer for 30 minutes. Stir in the cream or yogurt just before serving.

Pumpkin and Dill Seed Soup

2 lb. (1 kg.) diced pumpkin
2 tablespoons brown sugar
5 cups chicken stock
2 teaspoons dill seed
salt and pepper
1 teaspoon cinnamon
2 tablespoons fresh cream or yogurt

Put the pumpkin, sugar and a pinch of salt in a pan, cover with a little water, boil until the pumpkin is cooked. Drain off excess water, and put the pumpkin through a sieve or in the blender to make a purée. Return to the pan; slowly add the chicken stock, then the dill seed, stirring all the time; season with salt and pepper to taste. Simmer for 6 minutes, stir in the cinnamon; just before serving add the cream or yogurt.

Sorrel and Lentil Soup

¼ lb. (125 g.) lentils
7½ cups water
salt and pepper
1 cup sorrel leaves
2 tablespoons fresh cream or yogurt

Cook the lentils in the water for about 2 hours; put through a blender, adding a little more water if the purée becomes too thick. Return to the pan, season with salt and fresh pepper to taste. Chop the sorrel leaves, add them to the soup and simmer for 10 minutes. Just before serving the soup stir in the cream or yogurt.

Potato and Watercress Soup

4 potatoes

1 onion

2½ cups stock

1 bunch watercress

1 cup milk

1 tablespoon butter

3 egg yolks

salt and pepper

3 tablespoons grated cheese

Peel and chop the potatoes and onion; add to the boiling stock and simmer for ½ hour. Put through the blender. Finely chop the watercress for use later. Warm the milk and in it melt 1 tablespoon butter; beat the yolks and combine with the milk in the bottom of a serving dish. Return the soup to the heat, simmer until hot and add the chopped watercress for the final minute. Add a few spoonfuls of the soup to the milk-and-egg mixture, blend, pour in the rest, stir and season with salt and pepper to taste; sprinkle with grated cheese.

Tarragon Pea Soup

½ lb. (250 g.) dried peas

5 cups water

2 tablespoons fresh tarragon

2 teaspoons fresh cream

Boil the dried peas in the water until soft. Add the tarragon and simmer for a further 5 minutes. Put through a blender and stir in the fresh cream.

Gazpacho

4 tomatoes, peeled and chopped

1 large cucumber, diced

1 minced onion

1 green pepper, finely chopped

2 cups tomato juice

3 tablespoons olive oil

1 tablespoon cider vinegar

salt and pepper to taste

Mix all the ingredients in a bowl, blending the olive oil and vinegar into a dressing before adding. Refrigerate for several hours before serving.

Herb and Vegetable Soup

3 stalks celery

2 onions or 3 leeks

3 carrots

1 potato

3 tablespoons olive oil

7½ cups water

salt and pepper

1 small lettuce

2 cups spinach or sorrel leaves

½ cup mixed herbs – parsley, chervil, chives, marjoram and thyme are a good combination, all finely chopped

Chop celery, onions, potato and carrots; warm the olive oil and braise the celery and onions, then add the carrots and potato and braise all together for 10 minutes over low heat, with the pan covered. Add the water, salt and pepper to taste – a good amount of freshly ground black pepper is best. Bring to the boil and simmer for 10 minutes, or until the carrots are almost cooked. Chop the lettuce and spinach or sorrel and add to the soup together with herbs; simmer for a further 5 minutes.

Soupe au Pistou

1 onion
2 leeks (or another onion)
3 tablespoons olive oil
4 potatoes
$\frac{1}{2}$ lb. (250 g.) green beans
2 tomatoes
$7\frac{1}{2}$ cups water or stock
salt and pepper

For the pistou:
6 leaves fresh basil
2 cloves garlic
1 tablespoon olive oil
1 tablespoon Parmesan cheese

Chop the onion and leeks and sauté them in olive oil until soft. Chop the potatoes and beans, peel and chop the tomatoes. Add to the pan and cover with stock or water; season to taste, using freshly ground pepper. Cover and simmer for 40 minutes. Meanwhile make the pistou by crushing the basil and garlic together with the olive oil in a mortar; finally blend in the Parmesan cheese, very finely grated. Add the pistou to the soup just before serving.

Chilled Watercress Soup

1 lb. ($\frac{1}{2}$ kg.) potatoes
1 onion
$2\frac{1}{2}$ cups water
$2\frac{1}{2}$ cups milk
$1\frac{1}{2}$ cups finely chopped watercress leaves
salt and pepper
2 tablespoons fresh cream or yogurt

Chop the potatoes and onion, put in a saucepan with the water and simmer for $\frac{1}{2}$ hour. Put through a blender, return to the pan. Warm the milk in another pan and add it to the purée; toss in the cress, season and simmer over low heat for 5 minutes. Chill the soup well. Before serving stir in the cream or yogurt.

Sorrel Soup

$\frac{1}{4}$ lb. (125 g.) sorrel leaves
$\frac{1}{4}$ lb. (125 g.) margarine
1 lb. (500 g.) potatoes
$7\frac{1}{2}$ cups water
salt and pepper
2 egg yolks

Chop or shred the sorrel leaves; melt the margarine in a pan and stir in the sorrel, simmer until softened. Peel and chop the potatoes. Add water, potatoes and seasoning to the sorrel, bring to the boil and simmer for 40 minutes. Put the soup through a blender, return to the heat and slowly blend in the egg yolks, previously beaten. Do not boil. Garnish with parsley.

SALADS

Dandelion and Herbs

8 young dandelion leaves
½ lettuce
2 teaspoons fresh marjoram
2 teaspoons fresh mint
2 teaspoons chopped chives
4 tablespoons olive oil
1 tablespoon cider vinegar
1 clove garlic, finely chopped
1 teaspoon salt
freshly ground pepper

Break up the dandelion and lettuce leaves, tear the marjoram and mint into smaller pieces, add chives and mix altogether. Prepare the dressing from the remaining ingredients and pour over the salad at the last minute.

Cottage Cheese Salad

1 cup sliced radishes
1 cup diced celery
½ cup chopped green pepper
olive oil
vinegar
black pepper
1 cup cottage cheese
a little salt
a few chopped olives (optional)

Mix vegetables and keep in the refrigerator; prepare an olive oil, vinegar and pepper salad dressing, mix with the cottage cheese and then fold into the vegetables. Add salt to taste. A few chopped olives may be added for a garnish.

Piquant Zucchini

2 lb. (1 kg.) small zucchini
4 tablespoons chopped shallots
1 sweet red pepper, chopped
2 tablespoons chopped parsley
1 tablespoon chopped oregano
½ cup olive oil
3 tablespoons cider vinegar
1 teaspoon salt
freshly ground pepper
2 teaspoons honey
½ lb. (250 g.) pitted black olives

Slice the zucchini into rings, cook for 2 minutes in lightly salted boiling water; drain and leave to cool. Then add the shallots, red pepper, parsley and oregano. Make a dressing from the oil, vinegar, salt, pepper and honey – mix very well before pouring over the zucchini; garnish with the olives.

Fennel Salad

2 tablespoons olive oil
1 tablespoon cider vinegar
1 teaspoon salt
freshly ground pepper
1 large fennel bulb
10 pitted black olives
1 tablespoon chopped parsley

First prepare the dressing in the salad bowl, using the oil, vinegar, pepper and salt. Wash the fennel well, then slice into fine circles like onion rings. Toss well in the dressing and garnish with the olives and parsley.

Avocado and Chervil

2 ripe avocados
the juice of a lemon
1 teaspoon salt
freshly ground pepper
lettuce leaves to garnish
3 tablespoons chopped chervil

Slice the avocados lengthwise into thin strips; marinate in the lemon juice seasoned with salt and pepper; chill very well. Serve on a bed of lettuce, sprinkled with the chervil.

Turkish Cucumbers

1 clove garlic
2 cups yogurt
½ cup olive oil
4 cucumbers diced or sliced
lettuce leaves to garnish
chopped fresh mint

Crush the garlic and add it to the yogurt and olive oil; mix thoroughly and then fold in the cucumbers. Serve on a bed of lettuce leaves and sprinkle with chopped mint.

Onion and Tomato

3 medium-sized onions
3 tomatoes
half a cucumber
4 tablespoons olive oil
1 tablespoon cider vinegar
salt
freshly ground pepper
2 tablespoons chopped basil leaves

Thinly slice the onions, tomatoes and cucumber in rings. Mix the oil, vinegar and seasoning, and pour over the vegetables; garnish liberally with the basil. This salad needs to marinate for at least 30 minutes.

Cauliflower and Hyssop

1 small cauliflower
1 apple, chopped into small pieces
3 tablespoons finely chopped hyssop
2 cups yogurt
juice of half a lemon
2 teaspoons salt

Slice cauliflower flowerettes into small pieces, mix with the apple; add the hyssop, yogurt and lemon juice, and season with the salt. Toss well; serve chilled.

Tabbuleh

1 cup cracked wheat (also known as bulghar)
2 cups chopped parsley
2 tablespoons chopped white onions
½ cup chopped mint
2 cups chopped tomatoes
salt and freshly ground pepper
½ cup olive oil mixed with the juice of 3 lemons

Soak the cracked wheat in water for 30 minutes; drain well. Mix in all the other ingredients, adding the dressing last.

Lovage and Carrot

1 large carrot, finely grated

1 apple, grated

2 teaspoons finely chopped
    lovage

½ cup yogurt

1 tablespoon mayonnaise

1 teaspoon salt

lettuce leaves

1 white onion, peeled and sliced in
    rings

Mix together the carrot, apple, lovage, yogurt, mayonnaise and salt, but do it gently. Serve on the lettuce leaves and garnish with the onion rings and a few lovage leaves.

Fruit-flavoured Vegetable Salad

1 cup raw chopped carrots

1 cup chopped celery

1 cup chopped cabbage

½ cup diced apple

½ cup pineapple juice

The first four ingredients should be tossed together and covered with the pineapple juice; chill well before serving.

FISH

Herbal Bouillabaisse

1 small lobster

2 lb. (1 kg.) mixed fresh fish – haddock, halibut, flounder, whiting, shellfish, etc.

3 cloves garlic

2 large onions

2 tomatoes

1 cup olive oil

a sprig of thyme

a sprig of fennel

1 bay leaf

a strip of orange peel

a pinch of saffron

salt and pepper

a handful of parsley

Cut all the fish into small pieces, separating the coarse and delicate varieties. Crush the garlic, finely chop the onions and tomatoes and put in a heavy deep saucepan with the oil, herbs (but not the parsley), orange peel, saffron and seasoning. First add the coarser fish, cover with boiling water and cook for 5 minutes over a high flame. Add the remaining fish, and continue to cook fast for another 5 minutes. Remove from the heat; garnish with lots of chopped parsley.

Fish Fillets

8 fish fillets (any)

2 bay leaves

salt and pepper

½ cup white wine

chives

2 tablespoons butter

Roll the fillets and put in a lightly

oiled casserole with the bay leaves; season with salt and freshly ground pepper, pour over the white wine and sprinkle with chives; dab with the butter. Cook for $\frac{1}{2}$ hour in a moderate oven.

Marinated Trout
4 small trout
1 tablespoon olive oil
$\frac{1}{2}$ cup white wine
1 tablespoon honey
4 shallots, chopped
1 teaspoon cumin
salt and pepper
1 tablespoon chopped chives
chopped parsley

Make a marinade from the oil, wine, honey, shallots, cumin, salt and pepper; let the fish stand in this for an hour. Wrap each fish in foil, well oiled; put in a casserole and cook on a low flame or in a moderate oven for 40 minutes. Garnish with chives and parsley.

Fish Pie with Nuts and Herbs
2 cups cooked flaked fish
$1\frac{1}{2}$ cups béchamel, seasoned with salt, pepper and nutmeg
2 tablespoons chopped chives
1 tablespoon chopped walnuts
1 tablespoon chopped parsley
slices of lemon

Fold the fish into the béchamel sauce; put into a casserole and cover

with the herbs and nuts; cook in a moderate oven for 45 minutes; serve with lemon slices.

Tuna and Basil Mould
15 oz. (425 g.) can tuna fish
small can tomato purée
2 tablespoons chopped basil
1 tablespoon finely chopped onion
1 teaspoon ground ginger
$\frac{1}{4}$ cup hot water
2 tablespoons gelatine
8 oz. (225 g.) plain yogurt
salt and pepper

In a saucepan gently heat the purée, basil, onion and ginger; do not boil. Pour the hot water over the gelatine, mix until the liquid is clear and stir into the tomato mixture. Take from the heat; fold in the tuna and yogurt, season with salt and pepper. Pour into a mould and leave to set in the refrigerator. Additional fresh basil can be used as a garnish.

Broiled Fish with Fennel
For each person:
1 whole cleaned fish, e.g. whiting, small sea bass
salt and freshly ground pepper
1 small bunch green fennel
2 slices of lemon
olive oil

Wash and clean each fish; season with salt and pepper; on the upper side make four horizontal incisions. Broil the uncut side first; turn over and place lemon slices in alternate incisions and the ferny fennel sprigs in the other two, brush with a little olive oil; season with a little freshly ground pepper and place under the broiler until done.

Tarragon Fish Mould

1 lb. (500 g.) fish fillets
1 bay leaf
1 sprig thyme
1½ teaspoons salt
2½ cups apple cider
4 shallots
1 tablespoon chopped tarragon
1 small carton yogurt
½ lb. (250 g.) shrimps, shelled and chopped
2 tablespoons gelatine
¼ cup hot water

Put the fillets in a casserole, season with the bay leaf, thyme and salt. Pour over the cider, cover and bake in a moderate oven for 30 minutes. Drain and preserve the liquid stock. Finely flake the fish, discarding any bones; chop the shallots; add the fish, shallots, tarragon, yogurt and shrimps to the stock, stirring well; dissolve the gelatine in the hot water; stir into the fish mixture. Pour into a mould and leave to set in the refrigerator. Garnish with a sprig of tarragon and sliced stuffed olives.

Scallops in Chervil Sauce

6 tablespoons butter or margarine
1 lb. (½ kg.) scallops
2 level tablespoons wholewheat flour
1¼ cups chicken stock
2 tablespoons finely chopped chervil
2 teaspoons grated onion
salt and pepper to taste
4 oz. (120 g.) Gruyère cheese, grated
3 tablespoons dried breadcrumbs

Melt 2 tablespoons butter in a heavy skillet and braise the scallops for 3 minutes, constantly turning; drain. Melt the remaining butter, stir in the flour and add the chicken stock; stir constantly over a low heat until the sauce thickens, then add the chervil and onion; season with salt and freshly ground pepper. Take off the heat and mix in the scallops. Put into a casserole, cover with a mixture of cheese and breadcrumbs and bake in a moderate oven until the cheese melts.

POULTRY

Parsley Chicken

2 small chickens

1 large bunch parsley or 6 tablespoons dried parsley

2 tablespoons soft butter

$\frac{1}{4}$ cup soybean or sunflower oil

juice of $\frac{1}{2}$ lemon

2 cups chicken stock

salt and pepper

For the sauce:

2 tablespoons butter

2 tablespoons flour

1 tablespoon fresh chopped
tarragon

salt and freshly ground pepper

$\frac{1}{2}$ cup cream

Wash and dry the chickens. Finely chop the parsley and mix with the butter; put half into each chicken. Fasten any openings with skewers or by sewing. Heat the oil in a heavy casserole and brown the chickens quickly all over, without burning the skin. Reduce the heat and pour the lemon juice over the chickens; allow to stand for a minute before adding the stock and seasoning. Cook uncovered in a moderate oven for 40 minutes or until tender, basting every now and then. For the sauce, melt the butter and work in the flour; add the strained chicken stock from the casserole and stir; add the tarragon and simmer for a few minutes, reducing the liquid to a sauce consistency; season with salt and freshly ground pepper. Finally stir in the cream. Keep the sauce hot but do not allow it to boil. Pour over the chicken and garnish with parsley.

Tarragon Chicken and Broccoli Salad

2 chicken breasts

1 onion

1 carrot

1 celery stalk

salt and pepper

2 lb. (1 kg.) broccoli flowerettes

For the sauce:

1 tablespoon cider or wine vinegar

1 tablespoon chopped tarragon

$\frac{1}{2}$ cup sour cream

2 cups home-made mayonnaise

Skin, bone and divide the chicken breasts into two pieces; finely slice the onion, carrot and celery. Put into a pot, add just enough water to cover, with salt and pepper to taste; bring to the boil. Lower the heat, cover the pot and simmer until the chicken is tender. This should take about 8 minutes. Chill the chicken only in a covered container for at least an hour; then cut into small pieces. Meanwhile cook the broccoli in boiling water (minimum amount). This should take no longer than 5 minutes; it is important that the broccoli is firm. Drain and wipe dry. Chill for at least an hour. To make the sauce, combine the vinegar and tarragon and heat in a saucepan until the vinegar has evaporated; blend together the sour cream and mayonnaise, add the tarragon and mix well. Combine the chicken pieces, broccoli and sauce; chill covered for at least 6 hours or overnight.

Roast Chicken with Dill Sauce

1 roasting chicken
1 onion
4 sprigs fresh dill or 1 teaspoon dried dill seed
2 teaspoons soft butter
salt and pepper
$\frac{1}{2}$ cup dry white wine
1 cup chicken stock

For the sauce:
1 teaspoon cornstarch
1 teaspoon chopped fresh dill or $\frac{1}{2}$ teaspoon dried dill seed

Cut the onion in half and put inside the chicken together with the sprigs of dill. Smear the butter over the skin and season with salt and pepper to taste. Put in a roasting pan and add the wine and stock. Cook in a moderate oven for about an hour, basting every 10 or 15 minutes. Strain the liquid, put in a pan and bring to the boil. Mix the cornstarch with 1 tablespoon water, stir, pour in a little of the chicken liquid, blend well and return to the pan. Add dill, season to taste and allow to simmer for a few minutes until it has the correct consistency.

Spiced Rabbit

1 rabbit
$1\frac{1}{4}$ cups cider or wine vinegar
$\frac{1}{2}$ cup tomato pulp
2 stalks celery
10 chopped olives
1 tablespoon capers
4 tablespoons honey
salt and pepper

Cut the rabbit into small pieces, place in a heavy saucepan with all the ingredients, keeping the celery whole and stew the rabbit slowly for $1\frac{1}{2}$ hours or till quite tender. Adjust seasoning before serving, if necessary. This dish can be garnished with parsley or served with a dill or tarragon sauce (see Roast Chicken with Dill Sauce, above, and Tarragon Chicken and Broccoli Salad, p. 261).

Marjoram Chicken (boiled)

1 chicken
$1\frac{1}{4}$ cups water
juice of $\frac{1}{2}$ lemon
salt and freshly ground pepper
2 sprigs fresh marjoram or 2 teaspoons dried marjoram

For the sauce:
1 tablespoon cornstarch
a little milk
chopped marjoram

Place the chicken on a rack in a deep saucepan or casserole. Add the water, sprinkle the lemon juice over the chicken and season. Put the marjoram on the breast and tuck it into the wing and leg joints. Cover tightly and bring to the boil; turn the heat down very low and simmer gently for 2 hours. If it is to be eaten hot, remove the bird to a warm serving dish and make a sauce by thickening the stock with 1 tablespoon cornstarch mixed with a little milk; to this add a little chopped marjoram.

This dish can also be eaten cold; leave in the refrigerator overnight and the juice will gel; skim off the film of surface fat before serving.

Stewed Duck with Herbs

1 duck
salt and freshly ground pepper
1 sprig parsley
1 sprig thyme
small bay leaf
2 large onions
$\frac{2}{3}$ cup cooking brandy
$2\frac{1}{2}$ cups red wine (Bordeaux or Chianti)
1 tablespoon olive oil
4 strips bacon
1 garlic clove
8 oz. (250 g.) mushrooms

Cut the duck into pieces and put them in a heavy pot, season and add the herbs; slice the onions and put in the pot; pour over the brandy and red wine. Allow to marinate for at least 5 hours, preferably overnight.

In a fireproof casserole, heat the olive oil and slowly cook the bacon – do not allow the bacon to fry, but cook it enough for the flavour to permeate the oil and then remove the bacon. Heat the oil, put in the pieces of duck and brown for 10 minutes. Pour in the marinade; return the bacon to the pot; finely chop the garlic clove and the mushrooms and add to the dish; simmer very slowly for $1\frac{1}{4}$ hours. It is important to make sure that the duck is well browned and sealed before stewing.

Lemon Quail

For each person:
1 quail
$\frac{1}{4}$ lemon
2 teaspoons butter
salt and freshly ground pepper
sunflower or soybean oil
1 strip bacon

Clean the quail and squeeze a little juice from the wedge of lemon over the surface. Soften the butter and put it inside the quail together with the wedge of lemon; rub on the salt and pepper, brush with the oil and cover with a strip of bacon. Roast in a moderate oven until tender – about 20 minutes. This can be served with dill or tarragon sauce (see Roast Chicken with Dill Sauce, opposite, and Tarragon Chicken and Broccoli Salad, p. 261).

MEAT

Kidneys with Parsley and Wine

2 kidneys per person
2 teaspoons butter
1 bay leaf
salt and freshly ground pepper
2 teaspoons flour
½ cup white wine
½ cup chopped parsley

Cut the kidneys into thin slices; melt the butter in a pan and when hot, add the kidneys, bay leaf, salt and pepper; cook on a high heat for a few minutes, constantly shaking the pan and turning over the kidneys. The kidneys should be cooked in about 5 to 8 minutes. Sprinkle with the flour and stir it well into the surrounding liquid. Add the wine, return to the heat and simmer for a few minutes. Serve hot, sprinkled with parsley.

Lamb's Liver with Basil

1 lamb's liver
½ lb. (250 g.) bacon
2 tablespoons butter
2 tablespoons flour
2 tablespoons chopped basil
¼ cup red wine
1 cup stock

Slice the liver. Fry the bacon in its own fat until crisp, drain. In another pan, melt the butter. Dip the liver in the flour and cook for a few minutes in the heated butter, until it is brown on the outside and pink within; add the chopped basil and cover with wine and stock; simmer for a few minutes only. Arrange the liver, cooking liquid and bacon on a dish; garnish with a little freshly chopped basil.

Stuffed Eggplant with Oregano

2–3 large eggplants
4 tablespoons olive oil
1 chopped onion
2 garlic cloves, chopped
1½ lb. (700 g.) ground lamb or beef
1 lb. (500 g.) tomatoes, peeled and chopped
2 tablespoons tomato paste
2 tablespoons chopped fresh oregano or 1 tablespoon dried oregano
salt and freshly ground pepper
red wine to moisten if necessary
3 tablespoons grated Parmesan cheese

Wash and halve the eggplant. Heat the olive oil in a heavy pan and sauté the eggplant for 5 minutes on each side. Drain on brown paper. Put the onion and garlic in the pan, cook until soft, being careful not to scorch the garlic; add the meat, tomatoes, tomato paste, oregano, salt and pepper. Scoop the centres from the eggplant, chop and add to the other ingredients in the pan. Cook slowly until the mixture is well blended and soft. If it looks dry, add some red wine. Put the eggplant shells in a baking dish, and put the meat mixture into each one;

sprinkle with grated Parmesan and bake in a moderate oven until the cheese is thoroughly melted.

Herb Sausages
$\frac{1}{2}$ lb. (250 g.) finely ground pork
$\frac{1}{4}$ lb. (125 g.) ground pork fat
$\frac{1}{2}$ lb. (250 g.) finely ground veal
1 cup wholewheat breadcrumbs
1 grated lemon rind
$\frac{1}{4}$ teaspoon sage
$\frac{1}{4}$ teaspoon marjoram
$\frac{1}{2}$ teaspoon thyme
a grating of nutmeg
2 teaspoons salt
$\frac{1}{2}$ teaspoon freshly ground pepper

Mix together the meats and fat; blend in the remaining ingredients. Keep in the refrigerator overnight in a covered dish. Roll into sausage shapes and cook (without oil or fat) over a moderate heat, browning all over; make sure that they are cooked through.

Stuffed Cabbage Leaves with Bay
1 medium-sized cabbage
1 chopped onion
vegetable oil
1 lb. ($\frac{1}{2}$ kg.) ground beef
$\frac{3}{4}$ cup cooked rice
1 teaspoon crushed coriander seeds
salt and pepper
2 bay leaves
1 cup stock
2 teaspoons cornstarch
freshly chopped parsley to garnish

Cut the biggest leaves off the cabbage and cook for 5 minutes in lightly salted water. Drain well. Brown the onion in a little vegetable oil; combine it with the meat, rice, coriander seeds and seasoning. Mix well; put a handful of the mixture on each cabbage leaf, roll up carefully and secure with a toothpick if necessary. Place in a casserole with the bay leaves, pour in the stock, cover and simmer gently in a moderate oven for 45 minutes. Thicken the remaining liquid with a little cornstarch, pour this sauce over the stuffed cabbage leaves and garnish with parsley.

Tongue with Sweet and Sour Sauce
1 fresh tongue
2 onions, halved
1 carrot, sliced
2 stalks celery with leaves
6 sprigs parsley
salt and freshly ground pepper (or 8 peppercorns)

For the sauce:
$\frac{1}{2}$ cup brown sugar
1 tablespoon flour
4 teaspoons dry mustard
2 cups cream mixed with 2 beaten egg yolks
$\frac{1}{2}$ cup vinegar

Put the tongue with the onions, carrot, celery and parsley into a deep pot; cover with water; season with salt and pepper. Bring to the boil and simmer for about 3 hours, or until tender. Drain and preserve the liquid.

To make the sauce put $2\frac{1}{2}$ cups stock with the sugar, flour and mustard into a double boiler, blend well and gradually add the cream and egg yolk mixture; cook gently until it thickens and allow to cool. Stir in the vinegar before serving.

Veal with Tuna Sauce
2 lb. (1 kg.) chilled roast veal

For the tuna sauce:
3 egg yolks
salt
2 tablespoons olive oil
teaspoon lemon juice
2 oz. (60 g.) tuna fish

Make a stiff mayonnaise: beat the egg yolks with a pinch of salt, gradually add the oil, beating all the time, and finally stir in the lemon juice. Break up the tuna, mash very finely or put through a sieve; gradually incorporate it into the mayonnaise, blending until a smooth creamy texture is achieved.

Chill thoroughly. To serve, slice the veal finely and pour the tuna sauce over it.

Herb Meat Loaf
2 lb. (1 kg.) ground beef
1 cup wholewheat breadcrumbs
1 green pepper, finely chopped
1 onion, finely chopped
1 teaspoon French mustard
1 teaspoon soy sauce
$\frac{1}{2}$ teaspoon dried thyme
$\frac{1}{2}$ teaspoon marjoram
1 teaspoon dried sage
salt and pepper
2 beaten eggs
3 tablespoons vegetable oil

Mix thoroughly all the ingredients except the oil, adding the eggs last; moisten a loaf pan with a little oil and firmly pack in the mixture. Put in the refrigerator for at least an hour. Turn the loaf into a baking pan – it should come out easily – pour the vegetable oil over it and bake in a moderate oven for 1 hour. Serve with tomato purée (see page 250) to which has been added 1 tablespoon chopped marjoram.

VEGETABLES

Baked Eggs in Tomatoes with Basil
4 large firm tomatoes
4 tablespoons wholewheat
   breadcrumbs
2 tablespoons chopped basil

1 tablespoon chopped chives
salt and pepper
4 eggs
4 pieces hot wholewheat toast,
   lightly buttered

Cut the tops off the tomatoes, scoop out the insides and mash in a bowl. Add the breadcrumbs, basil, chives, salt and pepper to taste; blend into a firm paste, adding more breadcrumbs if the mixture is too sloppy. Break an egg into each tomato shell and cover with the breadcrumb mixture. Put in a baking dish and cook in a moderate oven until the tomatoes are soft but still retain their shape. This should take between 30 and 40 minutes. For serving, place the tomatoes on the toast and garnish with sprigs of basil.

White Beans with Herb Sauce

1 lb. ($\frac{1}{2}$ kg.) white beans

1 onion

2 crushed cloves garlic

1 tablespoon olive oil

1 lb. ($\frac{1}{2}$ kg) tomatoes (or 1 large can Italian plum tomatoes)

1 tablespoon honey

salt and freshly ground pepper

2 tablespoons chopped chervil

Soak the beans in water overnight. Simmer in lightly salted water for $1\frac{1}{2}$ hours or until soft. Drain. Chop the onion and sauté together with the garlic in the oil. Peel and chop the tomatoes and add to the pan together with the honey and seasoning. Cook for 10 minutes, stirring to make a purée. Add the beans, heat and add the chopped chervil 3 minutes before serving.

Marjoram Potato Pie

2 lb. (1 kg.) boiled potatoes

4 tablespoons butter

2 cloves garlic, chopped

2 tablespoons fresh chopped marjoram or 1 tablespoon dried marjoram

1 cup yogurt

Slice the potatoes; heat the butter in a heavy pan and sauté the garlic. Add the potatoes and cook until lightly browned. Sprinkle with marjoram and cook for a few more minutes. Transfer to a casserole, pour the yogurt over and bake in a moderate oven for 40 minutes.

Potato and Caraway Purée

1 lb. ($\frac{1}{2}$ kg.) potatoes

2 tablespoons butter or margarine

1 teaspoon caraway seeds

salt and pepper

$1\frac{1}{4}$ cups hot milk

1 egg yolk

1 tablespoon freshly chopped parsley for garnish

Boil the potatoes in their skins in lightly salted water; be careful not to overcook as they need to be firm; remove the skins and slice. Brown the slices in the butter or margarine over a medium heat, turning constantly. Then add the caraway seeds and salt and pepper to taste. Pour on the hot milk, cover and simmer over a very low heat for 15 minutes. The potatoes should be soft but not mushy or broken up. Combine the egg yolk with a few tablespoons of the hot liquid from the pan and stir into the liquid in the pan – turn off the heat while doing this to prevent curdling. Garnish with chopped parsley.

Braised Chicory with Marjoram

1 lb. ($\frac{1}{2}$ kg.) chicory
1 tablespoon chopped fresh mar-
    joram leaves or 2 teaspoons dried
    marjoram
salt and freshly ground pepper
2 tablespoons butter

Wash and trim the chicory, cut into thick rounds and put into a buttered casserole in layers with marjoram, salt, pepper and dots of butter on each layer. Bake in a moderate oven for $1 - 1\frac{1}{2}$ hours; the time of cooking depends on the quality of the chicory.

Fennel and Tomato Casserole

1 onion
3 cloves garlic
4 fennel bulbs
$\frac{1}{2}$ cup olive oil
1 large can Italian plum tomatoes
salt and freshly ground pepper
$\frac{1}{2}$ cup wholewheat breadcrumbs
3 tablespoons grated Parmesan
    cheese
grated rind of half lemon

Chop the onion and garlic, halve the fennel and cut it into wedges. Heat the oil in a heavy casserole; sauté the onions and garlic until soft and then add the fennel; cook until the fennel starts to brown, stirring from time to time. Now add the tomatoes and seasoning. Lower the heat and simmer for 5 minutes. Sprinkle with breadcrumbs, cheese and grated lemon rind; bake in a hot oven until the top is crisp – about 20 minutes.

Lentils and Curried Eggs

8 oz. (250 g.) lentils
2 onions
4 tablespoons butter
4 hard-boiled eggs
$1\frac{1}{2}$ tablespoons curry powder
$\frac{1}{2}$ cup hot water
salt and freshly ground pepper

Soak the lentils in water overnight. Slice the onions and sauté in the butter until golden. Prick the eggs all over with a fork, brush with about half of the curry powder and sauté with the onions for about 5 minutes; remove the eggs. Add the rest of the curry powder to the onions; mix well and slowly add the lentils. Cook for 5 minutes, stirring all the time. Add the hot water, salt and pepper. Replace the eggs, cover and simmer until the lentils are tender and have absorbed all the water – about 30 minutes.

Spiced Carrots

8 – 10 carrots
1 tablespoon butter
½ teaspoon mustard powder
1 tablespoon chopped parsley
½ teaspoon tarragon
salt and freshly ground pepper

Slice the carrots and cook in lightly salted water until just tender. Melt the butter in a pan; add a little water to the mustard and then blend into the butter; stir in the carrots, add the parsley and tarragon and season to taste.

Eggplant and Rosemary Casserole

1 large eggplant
2 tomatoes
1 onion
3 cloves garlic
2 teaspoons chopped rosemary or 1 teaspoon dried rosemary
1 tablespoon chopped parsley
1 tablespoon vegetable oil
salt and pepper

Slice the eggplant, cover with a little salt and leave for an hour – this draws the liquid out of the eggplant. Rinse under cold water and dry. Slice the tomatoes; chop the onion and garlic. In a casserole, arrange the eggplant, tomatoes and onions in layers with the garlic, herbs, seasoning and a little oil; finish with herbs and a smear of oil; cook in a moderate oven for an hour.

Baked Basil Tomatoes

1 lb. (½ kg.) tomatoes
2 onions
1 clove garlic
1 tablespoon chopped fresh basil
¼ cup wholewheat breadcrumbs
2 tablespoons butter
salt and pepper

Slice the tomatoes; finely chop the onions and garlic, but keep separate; put the tomatoes, onion, garlic and basil in layers in a buttered baking dish; sprinkle with breadcrumbs and dot with butter; season with salt and pepper and bake in a moderate oven for 20 minutes.

Baked Turnips

2 lb. (1 kg.) turnips
2 onions
2 cloves garlic
1½ cups milk
1 cup cream
salt and pepper
½ cup grated cheese
freshly chopped chives or parsley for garnish

Peel and slice the turnips; chop the onions; slice the garlic. Put all the ingredients except the cheese and parsley into a pan, bring to the boil and simmer for 3 minutes, stirring all the time. Grease a dish with a little butter, put in the mixture and cover with grated cheese. Bake in a moderate oven for 45 minutes. Serve garnished with freshly chopped chives or parsley.

Lettuce au Gratin
1 lettuce
1 tablespoon butter
1 tablespoon flour
$\frac{1}{2}$ cup milk
salt and pepper
$\frac{1}{2}$ teaspoon grated nutmeg
2 tablespoons grated cheese

Wash the lettuce; steam in a double boiler for 10 minutes. Drain and place in a casserole. Melt the butter in a small pan, add the flour and stir with a wooden spoon until smooth.

Slowly add the milk, stirring all the time, until it has the consistency of a thick sauce, and season with salt and pepper. Pour the sauce over the lettuce and sprinkle with the nutmeg and grated cheese. Brown in the oven or under the broiler.

Honeyed Carrots with Hyssop
6 carrots
2 tablespoons water
2 teaspoons honey
1 tablespoon finely chopped hyssop
salt and pepper

Cut the carrots into very thin slices, put in a pan with all the other ingredients and simmer over a low flame until tender.

FRUIT DESSERTS

Brandied Caraway Apples
6 apples
3 teaspoons caraway seeds
$1\frac{1}{2}$ tablespoons raisins
3 tablespoons clear honey
$\frac{1}{2}$ cup brandy or orange juice

Cut the apples in half, core them and place in a baking dish. Put some caraway seeds, raisins and honey in the centre of each half and pour the brandy or orange juice over and around the apples. Bake at 350°F (180°C) for about 45 minutes, or until soft, basting frequently during

cooking. Serve hot with cream or yogurt and the sauce from the pan.

Glazed Pears
4 large pears
2 teaspoons butter
2 teaspoons honey
1 teaspoon cinnamon
sugar syrup (1 cup water boiled with $\frac{1}{2}$ cup raw sugar or honey for 5 minutes)
1 cup of red or black currant jelly
angelica for decoration
cream or sour cream

Cut the pears in half and cut out the cores. Put a little butter, a $\frac{1}{2}$ teaspoon of honey and a pinch of cinnamon inside each pear hollow. Place them in a saucepan and pour over the sweet syrup. Cover and simmer slowly, basting from time to time, until just tender – this should take about 20 minutes. Add the fruit jelly and return to the heat for a few minutes; lift out the pears and pour the juice over; decorate each pear with an angelica stalk. Chill; serve with cream or sour cream.

Stuffed Melons

1 small melon per person
1 orange
1 grapefruit
any berries or fresh fruit in season, including some black or red ones to give colour to the dish
$\frac{1}{2}$ cup black or red currant jelly
$1\frac{1}{4}$ cups water

Cut off the tops of the melons to make a lid; remove the seeds and fibrous parts. Scoop out the rest of the melon in curly strips, but leave the skin firm and intact. Peel, clean and cut up the other fruits into segments or slices, but leave the berries whole. Mix with the melon strips and refrigerate. Put the currant jelly in a pan with the water, simmer for 5 minutes and then chill. To serve, fill the melon shells with the mixed fruit and

pour the currant juice over; put the lids back on.

Pineapple in Kirsch with Strawberries or Cherries

1 pineapple
2 tablespoons kirsch
1 pint (250 g.) strawberries (cleaned) or cherries (pitted and sliced)

Cut the base of the pineapple straight so it will stand; cut off the top and remove the inside – a long knife is necessary for this. Chop the pineapple into small chunks, put in a bowl with the strawberries or cherries; pour the kirsch over. Refrigerate for at least an hour; return the mixed fruit to the pineapple shell and replace the lid.

Melon and Ginger Sorbet

1 medium-sized melon
5 tablespoons soft brown sugar
4 tablespoons water
1 tablespoon ground ginger
juice of a lemon
2 egg whites
mint for decoration

Cut the melons in half and remove the seeds and fibrous matter. With a melon-baller scoop out little balls – about 12 or 15 – to be used to decorate the sorbet; put in the refrigerator. Cut up the rest of the melon, put in a pan together with the sugar, water, ginger and lemon juice. Cook over a low heat for 8 minutes. Remove the contents, put into a blender or food processor and blend until smooth. Refrigerate. Beat the egg whites until stiff and fold them into the melon purée just before it freezes. Return to the freezer until solid. Garnish with the fresh melon balls and a sprig of mint.

Poached Tangerines

6 tangerines
2½ cups water
2 tablespoons honey
1 stick cinnamon

Halve the tangerines, remove the pits; put the water in a large shallow pan and float the tangerines in it; the water must not cover the fruit. Drop a little honey on each tangerine half, add the cinnamon stick to the water and poach until the tangerine skins are very soft. The tangerines can be served hot or cold with cream or sour cream.

Grand Marnier Fruit Salad

2 pints (500 g.) strawberries
½ lb. (250 g.) peaches
¼ lb. (125 g.) green grapes
2 oranges
4 tablespoons Grand Marnier
1 tablespoon honey or brown
  sugar

Wash, hull and halve the strawberries; pit, peel and slice the peaches; remove the skin and pits from the grapes and cut in two; peel one orange, remove the pith and pits and cut into segments. Squeeze the other orange and add the juice to the Grand Marnier and honey (or brown sugar), mix very well and, if it is difficult to blend, put on a low heat, but only for a few minutes otherwise the Grand Marnier will evaporate. Mix the fruits together and pour the liquid over. Cool in the refrigerator for an hour before serving.

Banana and Lemon Sorbet

4 bananas
2 tablespoons honey
juice of 1 lemon
1 tablespoon dark rum
1 cup yogurt
2 egg whites
rind of 2 lemons
chopped nuts and cherries to
  decorate

Peel and mash the bananas, beat in the honey and add the lemon juice; blend in the rum; add the yogurt and mix to an even texture. Whisk the egg whites until stiff and fold into the banana mixture. Place in the freezer until half frozen; remove and then whisk again at the same time blending in the lemon rind.

Return to the freezer until completely frozen. Serve with a garnish of chopped nuts and cherries.

Apples in Cider
8 apples
¼ lb. (125 g.) raisins
1¼ cups sweet cider

Peel, core and slice the apples, put in a baking dish and sprinkle with the raisins; pour the cider over and bake for 30 minutes at 350°F, (180°C), basting from time to time. Dessert apples need no sweetening but if cooking apples are used, sprinkle them with a little honey or brown sugar before cooking.

PRESERVES

Apple Chutney
½ oz. (15 g.) mustard seed
15 apples
2½ cups cider vinegar
8 oz. (250 g.) brown sugar
2 oz. (60 g.) raisins
1 garlic clove
2 oz. (60 g.) onions
1 tablespoon dried chillies
1½ oz. (45 g.) powdered ginger
1 oz. (30 g.) salt

Wash the mustard seed in some extra vinegar and put in the sun or cool oven to dry. Peel, core and slice the apples and boil them with the vinegar and sugar until soft. Chop the raisins. Cut the garlic and onions into small pieces; cut the chillies into small pieces and grind them in a mortar, adding the ginger and mustard seeds. Add all the ingredients to the cooked apples, mix well and bottle when cold.

Candied Angelica
2 cups angelica roots and stalks
2 cups boiling water
¼ cup sea-salt
1 very green cabbage
1 cup water mixed with 1 cup cider vinegar
2 cups sugar
2 cups water

Put the washed angelica in a saucepan and cover with the boiling water and sea-salt; steep for 12 hours. Drain, peel and rinse in cold water. Put a layer of cabbage leaves in a clean pan, then a layer of angelica, then another of leaves, and so on, finishing with a layer of leaves on the top. Cover with the water-and-vinegar mixture. Boil slowly until the angelica becomes green; strain. Make a syrup from the sugar and 2 cups of water; add the angelica and cook for 20 minutes;

pour off and reserve the syrup. Put the angelica on a wire rack to cool for 2 days. Then once more boil together the syrup and angelica until the stalks and roots are candied. Drain on a rack until completely dry.

Carrot Jam

4 lb. (2 kg.) carrots
2 lb. (1 kg.) sugar
4 lemons
12 tablespoons margarine

Wash and grate the carrots, boil until reduced to a pulp, using as little water as possible. To every 1 lb. ($\frac{1}{2}$ kg.) pulp add $\frac{1}{2}$ lb. (250 g.) sugar, the juice and grated peel of 2 lemons and 6 tablespoons margarine. Boil for 1 hour.

Spiced Whole Grapes

2 lb. (1 kg.) seedless green grapes
1 lb. ($\frac{1}{2}$ kg.) raw sugar (brown)
$\frac{1}{2}$ cup cider vinegar
2 teaspoons mustard seed
1 teaspoon ground ginger
1 teaspoon ground allspice
2 bay leaves
1 oz. (30 g.) powdered fruit pectin

Wash the grapes; put the sugar and vinegar in a pan with all the herbs and spices, bring to the boil and simmer gently for 15 minutes, stirring from time to time. Remove the bay leaves. Add the grapes and pectin, bring to the boil again and simmer for 5 minutes, skimming away any scum. Remove from the heat, allow to stand for 15 minutes, stirring to avoid a skin setting on the top and bottle. Use within 4 weeks.

Indian Mint Chutney

1 cooking apple
1 small onion
4 tablespoons brown sugar
4 oz. (125 g.) fresh mint leaves
salt and cayenne pepper

Chop the apple into small pieces, put into the blender with all other ingredients and blend until a thick paste is formed. Chill in the refrigerator in covered jars. It is good with lamb and broiled fish.

Elderberry Ketchup

2 lb. (1 kg.) elderberries
2$\frac{1}{2}$ cups cider vinegar
1 oz. (30 g.) shallots or white onions
1$\frac{1}{2}$ oz. (45 g.) whole ginger
1 bay leaf
$\frac{1}{2}$ oz. (15 g.) peppercorns

Wash the berries and put in an unglazed or Pyrex casserole; boil the vinegar, pour over the berries and cook for 8 hours in a very cool oven. Strain, put into a pan with the onions or shallots, minced or cut very finely, peeled ginger, bay leaf and peppercorns. Boil for 10 minutes and allow to cool; remove the bay leaf; bottle.

Parsley Jelly

50 sprigs parsley
peel of 1 lemon
juice of 2 lemons
2 cups sugar

Wash the parsley and place in a saucepan with enough water just to cover, add the lemon peel and boil for about 1 hour. Strain; add the lemon juice to the liquid. Allowing a cup of sugar to a cup of the liquid, boil until it begins to set. Bottle and keep in a cool place. To be served with chicken or fish dishes.

Marjoram jelly can be made in the same way and served with any main course dish, or as a spread for toast and bread.

Elderberry Chutney

2 lb. (1 kg.) elderberries
1 large chopped onion
2 tablespoons brown sugar
1 teaspoon salt
2 teaspoons ground ginger
$\frac{1}{2}$ teaspoon mixed spices and cayenne
1 teaspoon ground mustard seed
$2\frac{1}{2}$ cups cider vinegar

Wash the berries well, put in a heavy pan and crush a little with a wooden spoon; add the chopped onion and all other ingredients. Slowly bring to the boil and simmer until it begins to thicken, stirring constantly all the time. Allow to cool before bottling.

Orange Marmalade with Coriander

4 oranges
2 lemons
6 cups water
1 tablespoon crushed coriander seeds
4 lb. (2 kg.) sugar

Keep the skin on the fruit, wash well and cut into slices; soak overnight in the water. Put the coriander seeds in a muslin bag, securely tied, and place in the pan with the fruit and water, bring to the boil and simmer until the peel is soft; add the sugar and boil until the liquid sets. The coriander gives the marmalade a very special spicy taste.

Rose Petal Honey

8 oz. (250 g.) whole roses (red or pink)
$3\frac{3}{4}$ cups boiling water
$2\frac{1}{2}$ lb. (1·25 kg.) liquid honey
juice and pits of 2 lemons

Select the scented opened petals of red and pink roses and cut off the white bases. Rinse well in cool water in a sieve; put in a bowl and pour over the boiling water; cover and leave standing for 6 hours. Strain – the liquid should be perfumed and pink. Pour the honey into a preserving pot, add the rose water, the lemon juice and the pits in a muslin bag. Bring to the boil, simmer for 30 minutes or until it sets; cool a little before pouring into jars.

Rose Hip Jelly

2 lb. (1 kg.) rose hips
approximately 2 lb. (1 kg.) sugar
2 or 3 lemons

The rose hips should be gathered before they go too soft; cut in half, put in a saucepan with enough water to cover; simmer gently until the hips are soft – usually under an hour. Strain and return to the pan allowing 1 lb. ($\frac{1}{2}$ kg.) sugar and the juice of 1 lemon to every $2\frac{1}{2}$ cups of the liquid. Simmer until the jelly sets. This jelly is good with poultry, game or fish dishes, and can also be used on bread.

Mint and Apple Jelly

6 lb. (3 kg.) apples
1 lemon
3 lb. ($1\frac{1}{2}$ kg.) sugar
30 sprigs of mint

Peel, core and slice the apples; place in a heavy pan with the juice and grated peel of the lemon; cover well with water and boil to a pulp. Put in a muslin bag and allow to drip for several hours (overnight is practical). Return the strained liquid to the pan, allowing 1 lb. ($\frac{1}{2}$ kg.) of sugar to every $2\frac{1}{2}$ cups juice; add the mint leaves and boil for 45 minutes; strain to remove all particles of mint and return to the heat for a few minutes until set. This

should be a delicate shade of green.

Spiced Apples

4 lb. (2 kg.) apples
1 quart (1 l.) cider vinegar
4 lb. (2 kg.) sugar
1 oz. (30 g.) cinnamon sticks
$\frac{1}{2}$ oz. (15 g.) cloves

Peel and slice the apples; in a pan boil together the vinegar, sugar and spices; simmer for 15 minutes, add the apples and cook until tender; take out the apples and put into jars; return the syrup to the heat and boil down until fairly thick; remove the spices; pour the syrup over the bottled apples.

Apple, Pear and Plum Jam

8 lb. (4 kg.) apples
8 lb. (4 kg.) pears
8 lb. (4 kg.) plums
juice of 1 lemon
$1\frac{1}{4}$ cups cider
$\frac{1}{4}$ oz. (7 g.) powdered cloves

Leave on the skins of all the fruits, cut into quarters and put into a heavy pan; add enough water to cover the base of the pan but not the fruit; bring to the boil and simmer until soft. Strain; return the juice to the pan, add the lemon juice, cider and cloves; boil quickly until thick enough to set.

BREADS

Wholewheat Herb Scones

1½ cups wholewheat flour

1 teaspoon baking powder

½ teaspoon salt

1 teaspoon raw sugar

4 tablespoons margarine

1 teaspoon mixed herbs (your
  choice)

5 tablespoons natural yogurt

Sift the dry ingredients into a bowl –
if the wholewheat flour is very
coarse, sift twice – and rub in the
margarine. Add the herbs and yogurt and mix until a soft dough is
formed. Form into flat ovals and
bake for about 25 minutes at 400°F
(200°C).

Basic Wholewheat Bread

6 cups wholewheat flour

1 tablespoon salt

½ cup vegetable oil

½ cup honey

2 cups warm water

½ oz. (15 g.) fresh yeast or 2 teaspoons dried yeast

Mix the flour, salt and oil in a large
bowl; in a separate bowl put the
honey, pour over the warm water
and blend in the yeast. (If dried yeast
is used, leave for 15 minutes to
activate.) Make a well in the flour
and pour in the yeast and honey
mixture. Blend until a firm dough is
formed. Knead on a floured surface
for about 10 minutes. Form a ball

with the dough, place in a covered
greased bowl and leave in a warm
place to rise for an hour – the dough
should double in size. Knead for
another 2 – 3 minutes; shape into a
loaf and put into a greased 2 lb.
(1 kg.) loaf tin; cover and leave until
it has reached the top of the tin.
Bake in a hot oven (450°F, 230°C)
for 10 minutes, then lower the heat
to 400°F (200°C) and bake for a
further 20 minutes, or until cooked
through.

Country Loaf

4 cups wholewheat flour

1 cup rye flour

1 cup cornmeal

1 tablespoon salt

1 cup milk

3 tablespoons water

2 tablespoons molasses

½ oz. (15 g.) fresh yeast or 2 teaspoons dried yeast

Mix the flours together with the salt;
in a saucepan combine the milk,
water, molasses and cook over a low
heat until the molasses has dissolved and is well blended. Put the
yeast into a bowl and slowly add the
milk and molasses, stirring to mix
thoroughly. Pour the yeast mixture
into the flours. Blend until a firm
dough is formed. Knead on a floured
surface for 10 minutes; put the
dough in a covered bowl, leave in a
warm place and allow to rise until it
has doubled in size. Knead for a few

minutes; make into two oval loaves and put on a greased baking sheet; make a couple of knife slits on the top; leave to rise again until about double in size; bake for 35 minutes at 400°F (200°C).

Coriander Cornbread

1 egg
$\frac{1}{4}$ cup vegetable oil
1 cup milk
1 cup plain wholewheat flour
1 cup finely ground cornmeal
3 teaspoons baking powder
1 tablespoon raw sugar
1 teaspoon salt
$\frac{1}{2}$ teaspoon ground coriander seeds

Beat together the egg, oil and milk; in another bowl mix together the dry ingredients and fold into the liquid mixture. Pour into a greased loaf tin and bake for 25 to 30 minutes at 375°F (190°C).

Wholewheat Pastry Crust

1 cup wholewheat flour
1 cup white flour
$\frac{1}{2}$ teaspoon salt
6 tablespoons margarine
4 tablespoons water

Sift the wholewheat flour twice, add the white flour and salt; rub in the margarine until the mixture is like breadcrumbs. Add the cold water (best if from the refrigerator) and mix into a dough. Roll out on a floured board. Put in greased pie tins and bake for 15 minutes at 355°F (180°C).

GRAINS

Nut and Grain Cereal

4 cups rolled oats
$\frac{1}{2}$ cup sunflower seeds
$\frac{1}{4}$ cup sesame seeds
$\frac{1}{4}$ cup ground coconut
$\frac{1}{8}$ cup wheatgerm
$\frac{1}{2}$ cup chopped almonds
3 tablespoons olive or sunflower oil
3 tablespoons honey

Mix together the dry ingredients and add the oil and honey; blend very well. Put into a baking tin and cook for 30 minutes at 350°F (180°C), but towards the end of the cooking time watch it carefully, as this cereal cake is inclined to burn. Serve with honey and milk as an alternative to packaged breakfast cereals.

Polenta

5 cups water
2 cups cornmeal
$\frac{1}{4}$ teaspoon grated nutmeg
salt and pepper

Put the water into a pan, add a pinch of salt and bring to the boil; stir in the cornmeal and simmer over a low heat for 20 minutes, stirring from time to time. When the polenta is thick, add the grated nutmeg and check the seasoning. Transfer the polenta to a baking dish; bake in an oven at 400°F (200°C) for 30 minutes, but check that it does not become too crisp. Ideally it should be served with game, but it goes well with any vegetable sauce.

Home-made Pasta

4 cups wholewheat flour or a mixture of wholewheat and white flour
1 teaspoon salt
4 eggs
2 tablespoons water

Mix the salt into the flour, then make into a mound on a large working surface. In a bowl, beat the eggs with the water. Make a hole in the mound of flour, pour in the egg mixture and with the hands bring the flour gradually into the liquid, kneading into a dough. A little extra water may be required to make it elastic. The kneading usually takes about 10 minutes. The dough can be wrapped in plastic wrap and stored in the refrigerator for 2 – 3 days. Roll out on a large floured surface. The dough can be cut into any size

strips – large oblongs for lasagne, noodle-width for fettucine, narrower for tagliatelle. After cutting, leave it in the air for an hour before cooking. Fresh pasta takes only 5–6 minutes to cook in boiling water – it will become very soggy if it is cooked any longer. It can be served with butter and grated Parmesan cheese or with basic tomato purée (see page 250) to which you can add any herb you like.

Barley and Mushroom Casserole

1 onion
1 garlic clove
2 tablespoons olive or corn oil
1 cup sliced mushrooms
8 oz. (250 g.) barley
salt and pepper
1 chicken stock cube
2½ cups water
2 bay leaves
2 tablespoons grated cheese, a strong variety

Chop the onion and garlic clove, heat the oil and sauté the onions and garlic for about 5 minutes; don't brown too much; add the sliced mushrooms and sauté for another minute. Add the barley and allow it to cook for about a minute, turning all the time. Add salt and pepper to taste. Put the mixture in a casserole. Meanwhile, dissolve the stock cube in the water, simmering for a few minutes; then pour over the barley mixture. Place the bay leaves on the top, but be sure they are submerged under the liquid; cover dish and leave overnight in a cool place. Bake the casserole for 45 minutes at 375°F (190°C); serve garnished with grated cheese.

Muesli

2 tablespoons rolled oats
4 tablespoons water
juice of ½ lemon
a little milk
2 tablespoons honey
2 tablespoons wheatgerm
fresh or dried fruit, nuts, yogurt
    (optional)

Soak oats overnight in water; in the morning add lemon juice, milk, honey and wheatgerm; mix well. Then add any fresh fruit – traditionally shredded apple – raisins, dried apricots, nuts and natural yogurt as you wish.

Gnocchi

4 oz. (120 g.) bread (preferably
    brown or wholewheat)
2½ cups water
1 egg
1 cup white flour or wholewheat
    flour
salt and pepper
grated nutmeg

Cut the bread into small chunks; put the water into a pan and heat,

adding the pieces of bread when tepid; simmer until all the water has been absorbed. Beat the egg, stir into the bread mixture, then add the flour. Stir well; if it is too solid add a little more water, but remember that this mixture has to be made into fairly solid balls. Season to taste and add a little grated nutmeg. Cover with a cloth and allow to stand for an hour. Sprinkle flour over a board or table; make the gnocchi mixture into little balls with the help of flour. When completed, allow to stand for about 10 minutes. Boil a pan of water, salt very slightly or add a chicken cube; drop in the gnocchi and boil fast but only for 5 minutes – if boiled any longer it will turn into a mush. Remove with a slotted spoon. Serve with butter and cheese, or with tomato purée (see page 250).

Boiled Brown Rice

2 teaspoons olive oil
8 oz. (250 g.) brown rice
2½ cups water
pinch salt

Heat the olive oil and pour in the rice, turning and cooking for a couple of minutes so that the rice is coated with oil. Add the water and a pinch of salt and bring to the boil; cover the pan, lower the heat and simmer for 30 to 40 minutes.

Risotto Milanese

6 teaspoons olive oil
1 onion
5 strips of bacon
8 oz. (250 g.) mushrooms
8 oz. (250 g.) rice
2½ cups vegetable stock (from any vegetable boiled in water)
salt and freshly ground pepper
4 tablespoons grated cheese, a strong variety
chopped parsley

Heat the oil in a heavy pan; chop the onion, bacon and mushrooms. Sauté the onion in the oil and, when it is beginning to brown, stir in the bacon; sauté for 5 minutes; put in the mushrooms and brown quickly for a minute. Add the rice, keeping the heat moderately high, and keep turning so that all the rice is coated with the oily mixture – this takes 1 – 2 minutes. Pour in the vegetable stock, stir and season. Bring to the boil, then turn down the heat and simmer for 15 minutes – the pot must be covered. Sometimes a little more water has to be added if the rice becomes too dry before being completely cooked. Add the grated cheese, stirring it in well. Serve garnished with chopped parsley.

Middle-Eastern Rice

2 tablespoons olive oil or corn oil
1 onion
8 oz. (250 g.) long-grain rice
4 oz. (120 g.) dried fruits, a mixture of raisins, apricots, pears or peaches, whatever is available
2 oz. (60 g.) walnuts
a pinch of cinnamon
sprinkling of grated nutmeg
2½ cups vegetable stock – from any vegetable boiled in water
salt and freshly ground pepper

Heat the oil in a sturdy pan; peel and chop the onion into small pieces; sauté for 5 minutes in the oil, only until lightly browned. Add the rice, the dried fruits, chopped or sliced, and the walnuts. Stir well, then add the cinnamon and nutmeg. Pour over the vegetable stock, stir and season. Bring to the boil, then lower the heat and simmer for 15 minutes or until rice is tender, but be sure not to overcook. At this point all the stock should have been absorbed. Finally put a cloth over the pan – a dish towel will do – and put the lid on; allow to stand for 10 minutes. Any excess moisture will be absorbed in the cloth, leaving the rice fluffy.

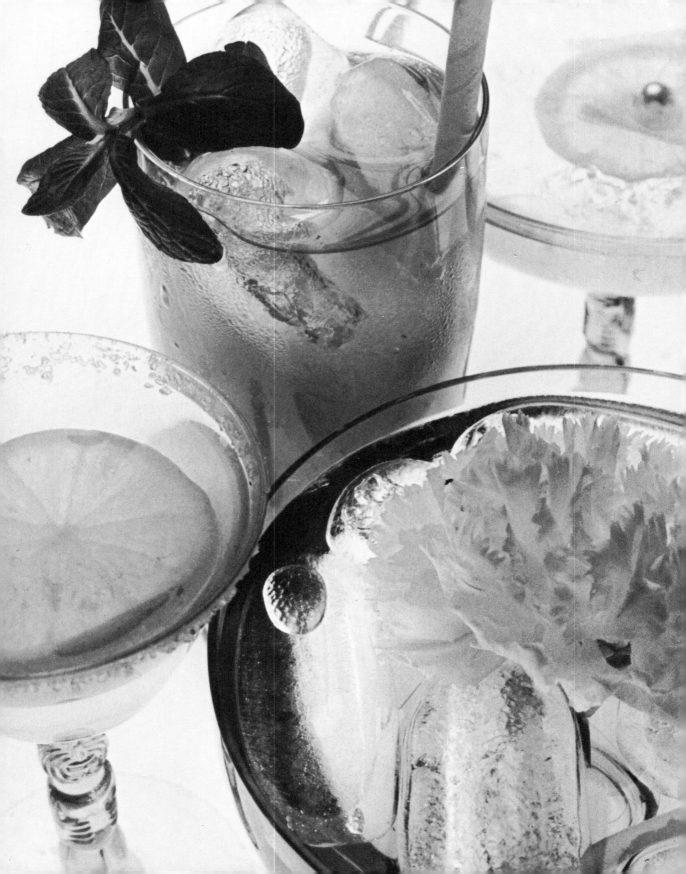

4

DRINKS

Although we eat primarily to appease hunger, we don't necessarily drink because we are thirsty. We also drink for stimulation.

Tea and coffee are mild stimulants and relatively harmless. Coffee contains caffeine which stimulates the brain and the nervous system; tea only has half as much caffeine but it is richer in theophylline which increases the heart rate and acts as a diuretic. Tea also contains a certain amount of fluorine which is good for the teeth. Both tea and coffee are a source of vitamin B-3 and some vitamin B-1 and B-2. Cocoa has some stimulants too but they are less apparent as the body does not readily absorb them.

The most natural alcoholic stimulant is wine. Taken in moderation it is beneficial for it contains many minerals and vitamins, as well as enzymes that aid in the digestion of food. Alcohol is quickly assimilated and dilates the blood vessels, which explains why it is sometimes prescribed in moderation for circulatory troubles. It also depresses the centres of anxiety and can therefore be an aid to relaxation.

Wine provides vitamins B-2, B-3, B-5 and B-6, also small quantities of B-1, B-12 and folic acid. Minerals present are magnesium, calcium, sodium, potassium and phosphorus. Dry red wine is a good source of iron. Anti-bacterial elements are present and by drinking wine we indirectly draw energy from the sun. The vitamin and mineral content of a wine depends on the soil and climate in which it was produced. A French homoeopathic physician, Dr E. A. Maury, has done extensive research into the medicinal value of wines; in his book *Wine is the Best Medicine* he gives details of the composition of wine and which wines can help specific diseases. He concentrates on wines of French origin, claiming comforting facts such as that champagne is good for certain liver complaints and heart disease, Loire wines break down cholesterol and Graves wines are good for anaemia because of their high iron content.

Natural wines are healthy, but many commercial wines are doctored with chemicals to quicken maturity, clear away sediment or enable them to travel better. As to the actual alcoholic content, ordinary table wines have no more than 10 to 12 per cent alcohol. Wines are carbohydrates; the sweeter or heavier the wine, the more sugar elements it contains.

The making of wine is a completely natural process, as the grape contains the necessary sugar and natural yeasts. Wine can be made from the fermented juice of any fruit, but either sugar or yeast or both have to be added. The crushing of the grapes begins the process. White wine is made from white grapes, black grapes or a combination of both, since only the colourless flesh and juice are left to ferment. For red wine, only black grapes are used and the skin is present during fermentation. Rosé wine is made by leaving some skins with the juice. Sparkling wines and champagnes are produced by bottling the wine before fermentation has finished so it retains some of the natural carbon dioxide which is produced.

Spirits and liqueurs are more concentrated alcohol and are distilled from original wines or fermentations of other fruits and grains. Their main effect is stimulation; they may in fact take vitamins away from the body because, like any sugar carbohydrate, they cannot be assimilated without the vitamin B complex. Dry spirits such as whisky, white rum, vodka and gin have less sugar content than sherry, port, vermouths and the sweet liqueurs.

Healthy drinks are not difficult to make; they fall into four categories: teas, milks, vegetable and fruit juices, wines. (For details of herbal teas refer to pages 120–32; for fruit and vegetable juices and their value see pages 16–19.)

TEAS

Mint Tea

For a refreshing tangy drink, add a teaspoon of dried peppermint leaves to the tea in the teapot. Try peppermint leaves with fresh coffee too.

Spiced tea

2 tablespoons tea (any variety)
1 stick cinnamon
2 cloves
5 cups boiling water

juice of 1 lemon
juice of 1 orange
slices of lemon or orange

Mix together the dry ingredients, pour the boiling water over and add the lemon and orange juice; cover and steep for 5 minutes; serve with slices of lemon or orange.

Nightcap Tisane

1 oz. (30 g.) dried peppermint leaves

1 tablespoon fresh rosemary (or ½ tablespoon dried)

1 teaspoon chopped fresh sage (or ½ teaspoon dried)

Mix well together and use 1 good

teaspoon to a cup of boiling water; allow to infuse for a few minutes; sweeten the drink with honey if necessary.

Slimming Tisane

equal parts of:
verbena
thyme
mallow
sage
orange blossoms

Mix well and use 1 heaped tablespoon to a cup of boiling water; infuse for 5–10 minutes. No sweetening.

MILKS

Extra-protein Milk

1 egg yolk

1¼ cups milk

2 teaspoons peanut or olive oil

1 tablespoon wheatgerm

1 teaspoon honey

Beat the egg yolk into the milk and slowly add the other ingredients; it is more easily done in a blender.

Carrot Milk

½ cup carrot juice

½ cup milk

½ lemon or orange (optional)

Beat together the carrot juice and milk; add the juice of half a lemon or orange for a tangy taste.

Raspberry Milk

2 tablespoons blackberry juice

2 tablespoons raspberry juice

½ cup milk

1 teaspoon honey

1 teaspoon dried lemon balm

Mix all the ingredients in a blender, leave to stand for 30 minutes, then refrigerate and serve chilled.

Orange-Apple Milk

¼ cup orange juice

¼ cup apple juice

½ cup milk

1 teaspoon honey

1 teaspoon dried sweet cicely

1 teaspoon lemon juice

Mix all the ingredients in a blender. Cover and leave to stand for 30 minutes. Put in the refrigerator and serve when chilled.

Fortified Milk

5 cups fresh skimmed milk

1 cup dried milk (skimmed)

2 tablespoons olive or sunflower oil

Mix thoroughly in a blender to make a basis for adding other ingredients: 1 tablespoon carob powder, which gives a chocolate flavour; $\frac{1}{4}$ teaspoon powdered nutmeg; $\frac{1}{4}$ teaspoon powdered cinnamon; 2 tablespoons molasses; a few drops of vanilla or 2 teaspoons of instant coffee.

Elder Flower Milk

1 bunch of elder flowers or 1 tablespoon dried elder flowers

1 teaspoon freshly chopped or dried lemon balm

$\frac{1}{2}$ cup milk

1 teaspoon honey

Heat the milk, but do not allow it to boil, and pour over the elder flowers and lemon balm. Steep for 10 minutes. Strain, add the honey and mix well. Serve chilled.

JUICES

Fruit Juice Yogurt

1 cup yogurt

1 tablespoon of any frozen fruit juice (unsweetened)

1 teaspoon honey

Mix together.

Caraway Tomato Juice

1 cup tomato juice

1 cup cabbage juice

3 tablespoons brewer's yeast

1 teaspoon caraway seeds

Crush the caraway seeds, then mix all ingredients in a blender; serve chilled.

Super-Health Drink

2 cups yogurt

$\frac{3}{4}$ cup milk

3 tablespoons freshly chopped spinach

1 tablespoon tomato paste

2 teaspoons wheatgerm

1 teaspoon brewer's yeast

2 egg yolks

1 teaspoon ground almonds

juice of 1 lemon

juice of 1 orange

1 tablespoon chopped parsley

Mix all together in a blender until thoroughly liquidized. Chill before drinking. It can be taken as a cocktail or in between meals; it can actually substitute for meals for a three-day diet régime as it contains protein, vitamins and minerals.

Apple Juice Plus

1 cup apple juice
1 tablespoon dried milk (skimmed)
5 walnut kernels or 1 tablespoon ground almonds
1 teaspoon wheatgerm
1 teaspoon brewer's yeast
1 teaspoon honey
strawberries, banana or black currants (optional)

Mix the first six ingredients together in a blender; for extra flavour another fruit can be added – strawberries, banana, black currants, etc.

Spiced Tomato Tea

1 cup tomato juice
4 tablespoons brewer's yeast
1 tablespoon lemon juice
1 tablespoon chopped parsley
$\frac{1}{2}$ tablespoon chopped chives

Mix together in a blender; refrigerate and cool before drinking. This can serve in the place of a cocktail.

Yogurt and Tomato

$\frac{1}{2}$ cup tomato juice
$\frac{1}{2}$ cup yogurt
1 teaspoon lemon juice
pinch sea- or vegetable salt

Mix everything together.

WINES

Coltsfoot Wine

20 cups water
3 lb. (1·4 kg.) sugar
$\frac{3}{4}$ oz. (20 g.) fresh yeast or 1 tablespoon dried brewer's yeast
2 oranges
2 lemons
10 cups coltsfoot flowers

Warm the water and dissolve the sugar in it; remove from heat and cool. Pour a little of this liquid onto the yeast and leave to activate. Peel the oranges and lemons and cut the rinds into strips; extract the juice from the fruits; put the peel, juice and flowers into an earthenware jar; pour the sugar syrup over and stir. Add the yeast mixture and leave to ferment in a warm place, covered with a cloth for 5 – 6 days, stirring daily. When the fermentation subsides, strain it into jars and cover with plastic wrap. When the fermentation stops, bottle.

Dandelion Wine

10 cups stripped dandelion petals
20 cups water
3 lb. (1·4 kg.) sugar
1 lemon
1 orange
1 tablespoon brewer's yeast

Strip the petals from the dandelion flowers. Boil the water and pour over the petals; cover and allow to infuse for 10 days, stirring occasionally. Strain the liquid; put into a preserving pan and add the sugar. Grate the rind from the lemon and orange, cut up the flesh, removing pits and any trace of white skin; add the rind and fruit chunks to the liquid; boil gently for 20 minutes; cool until tepid then add the brewer's yeast. Cover with a cloth and allow to ferment for 2 days. Put into a deep earthenware bottle or cask and cover with plastic wrap; check the fermentation and when it stops, bottle. This takes about 2 months.

Cassis

1 cup black currant juice
1 bottle dry white wine
2 bottles soda water
1 lemon, sliced

Stir the black currant juice into the wine; allow to stand for an hour; add the soda water and lemon just before serving. Particularly good over crushed ice.

Rosemary Wine

4 cups white wine
2 tablespoons chopped fresh rosemary

Pour the wine over the rosemary, cover and infuse for 2 days. Strain. Drink as an aperitif or tonic in sherry glasses.

Spiced White Wine

10 cups white wine
8 oz. (250 g.) brown sugar
1 teaspoon cinnamon
5 tablespoons chopped marjoram leaves
2 peppercorns
$\frac{1}{2}$ lemon, sliced

Put all the ingredients in an earthenware container; cover and allow to stand for 5 hours. Strain, chill and serve.

Mulled Wine

$2\frac{1}{2}$ cups red wine
2 tablespoons brown sugar or honey
1 teaspoon cinnamon
6 cloves
grated peel of 1 lemon

Heat the red wine, add all the other ingredients and bring almost to the boil; cover and allow to stand for 5 minutes. Strain. Add a slice of lemon to each glass, serving the wine hot. A good bedtime drink.

Elderberry Wine

½ oz. (15 g.) ginger
6 cloves
20 cups water
20 cups elderberries
1 lb. (½ kg.) raisins
3 lb. (1·4 kg.) brown sugar

Put the spices in the water and boil for ½ hour. Add the elderberries and raisins, return to the heat and boil again for 30 minutes. Allow to stand until completely cold, then stir in the sugar until all is thoroughly blended. Cover and leave in a cool place for 1 month. Strain before bottling; leave for 6 months before drinking, but always keep bottled wine in a cool place.

Rose Cup

2½ cups water
5 oz. (150 g.) red rose petals
2½ cups brandy
1 cup sugar
1 teaspoon cinnamon
1 teaspoon coriander seeds

Heat the water until it is a little warmer than tepid, pour over the rose petals and steep for 2 days in a covered pot. Strain. Stir in the brandy, add the sugar, cinnamon and crushed coriander seeds. Cover and steep for 2 weeks; strain and bottle. Drink as an aperitif.

Srawberry Cup

2 sprigs each of sage, mint and lemon balm
2 bottles white wine
2 pints strawberries
1 tablespoon sugar
2 bottles soda water

Chop and crush the herbs (if dried use a good tablespoon of each – fresh is better). Put the herbs into an earthenware pot, pour over the wine, cover and leave to stand for 3 – 4 hours; strain. Cut the strawberries into halves, sugar lightly and drop into the liquid. Just before serving add the soda water.

Claret Cup

1 tablespoon sugar
2 tablespoons hot water
1 bottle red Bordeaux wine
rind and juice of 1 lemon
1 glass sherry
1 teaspoon grated nutmeg
1 tablespoon chopped fresh or dried lemon verbena
1 bottle soda water
3 sprigs borage

Dissolve the sugar in the hot water, add the next six ingredients, stir well, cover and leave to stand for 1 hour; strain. Chill in the refrigerator before serving, and decorate with sprigs of borage.

INDEX